JOURNEY TO MASTERY

Feng Shui for Life

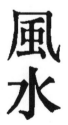

by
Dr. Kathryn Mickle, Ph.D.
Wellness Institute for Research and Education

First Edition
©Copyright 2001 by Dr. Kathryn Mickle, Ph.D.
Published by Frederick Fell Publishers, Inc.
2131 Hollywood Blvd., Suite 305, Hollywood, Florida 33020
www.fellpub.com

Printed in the United States of America.

ISBN 0-88391-025-x

CONTENTS

CONTENTS *continued*

Acknowledgements

Thank you to my good friend and supporter, Kitty Oliver, who has been there always, encouraging me through the writing process and acting as a friendly reader.

Thank you to my mentor, Michael Harris of *Peter Lowe International* for his inspiration and guidance, helping me to stay focused on this book.

Thank you to Sean Jones for the artistic cover design and book setup and to Douglas Schules and Dr. Jacklyn Neblett for their arduous editing.

Along my spiritual path, there have been beacons which have helped my understanding. Among these are:

The Orin and Daben Writings by Sanaya Roman and Duayne Packer,

The Course in Miracles,

The Kryon Writings by Lee Carroll and *Indigo Children* by Lee Carroll and Jan Tober.

There are many teachers along my Eastern path who filled in pieces of the puzzle for me. These include:

Master Mantak Chi
Master Dannie Wu
Raven Merle
Michael Andron

I would like to acknowledge my husband, Van, whose constant provoking made me look more closely at my patterns and Trinidad and Tobago, his homeland, where I found the peace to write large parts of this book.

Forward

Jami Lin

I liked her immediately. Through professional association and a co-operative educational Feng Shui group in which we are founding members, I have come to respect Kathryn's knowledge, professionalism, dedication, and integrity. When she asked me to write her foreword, I was delighted. I thought, now I can really get to know her while at the same time have opportunities to possibly learn something new, perhaps explore life with a different approach, and most definitely, be reminded to focus on my inner journey.

As I read, the more beautiful Kathryn became. I saw her knowledge and experience, as well as her gentle, kind, and loving approach. With or without you having an education in Feng Shui, basic physiological understanding, knowledge about Eastern practices, Dr Mickle, my friend and colleague, delivers. She provides easy to apply principles to get to know yourself better, thus helping you to improve the quality of your life.

Often sharing her life obstacles, her journey to mastery reminds us that with each passage there is always more to learn. She reaffirms that we all, no matter what life presents, have similar universal needs. Most importantly, she helps us to remember what aspects truly help us live with happiness and joy. Knowing that life sometimes appears to throw us a curve, she provides us with loving-our-self tools that we can use to graciously recognize blockages and to easily meet the challenges.

Kathryn's innovate approach uses the ancient Chinese Bagua, which defines the energetic workings of the cosmos, the planet, the seasons, and even the structure of family. As your life journey evolves, she describes Bagua concepts as a guide to understanding, guiding the enhancement of your life. Through the basics of

Chinese metaphysics we are all reminded of many living skills including to:

° Be kind and loving to ourselves in order to be kind and loving to others
° Be conscious and observant of our bodies and thoughts
° Replace negative thoughts with those that are positive
° Live in the here and now instead of the past or future

With Kathryn's well written and enjoyable book, we are encouraged to always journey through the cycles of life, year by year, day by day, and minute by minute, as we all share the birthright to celebrate life and its mastery.

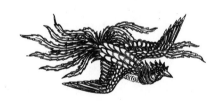

Introduction

In the early eighties, while I was living in Toronto, Canada doing my Ph.D. research, I chose to study how students from other cultures dealt with the stress of adapting to a new society. As I looked over the student population, the students from Hong Kong were, statistically, the easiest group to study. At that time, because of the fear of the takeover by mainland China in 1997, families from Hong Kong were sending their children to North America, as well as to England and Australia, to create homes outside the country. These students were very stressed because they were under tremendous pressure from their families to do well at school and often had to cope with courses that were not their choice as well as a new language and culture.

I had several hypotheses about conditions that I felt would lessen the impact of stress, but what became very apparent to me was that I had not taken into account these students' practices. I learned from them that many of them used T'ai Chi Ch'uan (also known as T'ai Chi and Taijiquan), Qigong (Chi Kung), and Feng Shui as well as the accompanying philosophy, to help them deal with upsetting situations. The ones who utilized these practices were able to handle the pressures of adapting to a new society much more effectively.

A little while later, I realized the power of these practices myself. After receiving my doctorate, I was working full-time in an administrative position and doing part-time teaching at a university. I had also opened a clothing store and, through it, was involved in a direct sales company. As well, I was a recently divorced mother of two boys. As you can well imagine, I was under a lot of stress myself. My way of stress reduction was to do dance aerobics, swim or play tennis. It was after an injury, caused by these strenuous activities, that I discovered T'ai Chi Ch'uan for myself. I found that the slow, gentle movement had a calming effect on me and gave me more energy, resilience and strength in my body.

At the same time, I also had a part-time practice as a psychotherapist, helping people deal with life's problems and the emotions accompanying them. I had been using psychotherapy and cognitive methods to help people deal with emotional turmoil and stress but had never thought of incorporating Eastern practices into my therapy. As I did these practices myself, I realized that adding them to my counseling would make it more effective.

Over the years, I have modified my methods of therapy. Now I use a mixture of counseling, hypnotherapy, Eastern practices and philosophy. Hypnotherapy helps us release conditioned thinking patterns which have been with us from childhood. The practices of Qigong, T'ai Chi Ch'uan and Feng Shui, with their emphasis on balance and harmony, along with the underlying Taoist philosophy, teach people a calmer way of dealing with strong, emotional situations. Properly understood, Eastern practices can be an effective therapeutic tool.

The use of these practices became even more important to me when I was trying to sell my house. The majority of house buyers in Toronto were immigrants from Hong Kong. I was told by my real estate agent that these people would not consider my house because it had bad Feng Shui. At that time, I did not know what that was but I did know that I had bad luck in that home. My first marriage ended in divorce and I had financial setbacks while living there. I finally sold it to non-Chinese buyers. Later, when I began to study Feng Shui, I realized that there were many things I could have done to cure different areas in my house to change the energy of my living space and my life.

In this book, Feng Shui shall be used as a model to change the energy of your life. Also I will introduce concepts that I have found helpful from Qigong and T'ai Chi, the philosophy of Taoism, and from my long association with many Chinese people. I blend these concepts with modern psychological tools to help you analyze your life and to help you achieve mental, physical and spiritual wellness, which I call mastery.

Feng Shui

The concept of Feng Shui is associated mainly with the Chinese. However, it may have had its roots in India and Tibet, evolving into agrarian China where harmony with the natural surroundings was of primary importance. Originally it was called "Kan Yu," which means heaven and earth. This name shows the ancient Chinese view that the unseen world influenced the manifested world. The words "Feng Shui" mean wind and water, which, according to the ancient Chinese, are the main intermediaries between heaven and earth. It evolved into a practical study of the energetic principles of the earth, looking at how to best tap the vitality flowing into any environment. It was used later to come up with the most auspicious burial spots for ancestors so that the descendants' luck would continue for generations.

In modern times, this art is used to enhance aspects of life such as business, prosperity, health and luck by moving and placing things so that the energy will flow smoothly, without creating any blockages.

There are many ways of practicing Feng Shui. Some rely on direction and others do not. There are some in which the placement of objects changes according to the year and to your particular horoscope.

Many of you who have been introduced to Feng Shui may have become confused by the different methods. Which one is right, you wonder? The most important thing to remember is that all these methods have one thing in common: stimulating the best use of energy in your environment. You place objects in a certain way and combine shapes and colors to create harmonious surroundings.

Let us take a closer look at this. Man's relationship with his environment is an intimate one. Instinctively we know whether we would like to spend more time in some places. There is a spirit which can be felt intuitively, not perceived through our five senses. When we live or work in a place, we create our environment by introducing symbols which represent who we are. Our external and internal worlds are a reflection of one another, a fact well known by indigenous tribes for centuries but only recently being discovered by our modern world.

Feng Shui

Feng Shui is one of the Eight Branches of Chinese Medicine. The other branches include self-cultivation and meditation, movement such as Qigong and T'ai Chi, nutrition, bodywork and massage, cosmology and philosophy, herbal medicine and acupuncture. They all have in common the same concepts: Tao, Qi (Chi) or energy, the theory of Yin and Yang, the five elements, and the bagua (also spelled ba gua and pa kua).

Tao

Tao is hard to define. The opening chapter of the *Tao Te Ching* reminds us that the Tao that can be told is not the real Tao. It is nameless but refers to the eternal way or path. The classical definition is closest to universal life force or our concept of God.

Qi (Chi)

We recognize now that we live in a world of energy and vibration. This invisible energy called "qi" (chi) by the Chinese, "ki" by the Japanese and "prana" by the Yogis flows constantly though all life forms. Modern medical practices recently have observed this energy movement flowing through the body in the seven energy chakras and in the acupuncture meridians. The earth has similar meridians called ley lines and other spots of incredible energy where ancient civilizations erected their temples and monuments.

Like Qigong and T'ai Chi, which enhance the flow of energy in our bodies, Feng Shui is an art which stimulates the optimal flow of energy through our environment. It has been likened to the acupuncture of the environment. The cultivation of qi, in these physical practices, refines the energies of our mind and body so that we can access the energy of Spirit. Some practitioners of Feng Shui believe that a change can take place only through the use of esoteric and transcendental solutions, which access the unseen world beyond the five senses. I believe that, for us to grow to mastery, we must also deal with this unseen world.

Yin and Yang

The understanding of Yin and Yang is crucial to Feng Shui. They refer to two qualities of universal force energy or qi, and are represented as the positive and negative poles. They are inseparable tendencies of this energy and cannot exist without each other. All energy and material forms have these positive and negative polarities, just as electricity has a positive and negative charge. Yin and Yang are opposing polarities but are, in fact, complementary. For example, dark is yin and light is yang. Mountains and valleys are passive and yin; rivers and lakes are active and yang. The moon is yin and the sun is yang. For our environment to be balanced, we need to have both of these qualities equally represented.

The Five Elements

The Taoists observed that Yin and Yang interactions followed five basic patterns or five phases, which have been translated as the five elements. The physical elements found in nature symbolically express the motion of these five processes of energy. Each one is associated with a season. The energy of water represents energy sinking, like water submerged under ice in winter, the season associated with this element. Energy expanding or sprouting, like in the spring, is wood. Energy rising or sustained at its highest level is fire, like the season of summer. Energy solidifying or contracting after being sustained at a high level, like the season of fall, is metal. And stable energy, like the soil under our feet, is earth, which, like the season of Indian summer, provides a hiatus between late summer and fall. These elements also describe the sun's daily pattern. It rises in the morning (wood or East), is at full strength at noon (fire or South), wanes in the afternoon (earth or Southwest), sets in the late afternoon (metal or West) and is hidden at night (water or North). These elements and directions are represented in the eight-sided figure, the bagua.

The Bagua

A map called the bagua is placed over a lot, house or room to determine the optimal placement of objects and symbols for the harmonious flow of energy. Even though there have been indications that it may have existed before then, the bagua, as we know it, emerged from the I Ching, called the Book of Changes, which has its history in ancient China approximately 3000 years ago. Supposedly it was originated by the sage Fu Hsi, who was meditating on the bank of a river and was inspired by the markings on the back of a turtle emerging from the water. He saw that the whole universe was represented in these orderly markings.

He saw configurations of solid and broken lines, arranged in threes, in all possible combinations. Fu Hsi assigned the value of Yang to the solid line and Yin to the broken line. These groups of three, called trigrams, symbolized all aspects of nature: Heaven, Earth, Fire, Mountain, Lake, Deep Water, Wind and Thunder. These trigrams make up an eight-sided figure or octagon which is called the bagua.

Using the Bagua

Picture this octagon fitting, like a map, over your house, your lot, your room and even a smaller space; for example, your desk. These eight sides represent all areas of your life, all the Chinese elements and even your body. If you look at a human's body from the front, you will see that the organs are set up as a bagua, with the heart at the top (representing fire), the kidneys (water element) at the bottom, the liver (wood) on the left side, the lungs (metal) figuratively on the right, and the spleen in the middle (representing earth).

Another interpretation of the bagua notes that these trigrams represent the archetype of a family and links these family members with an element. In this system, the family is as follows: mother (earth), father (metal), oldest son (wood), second son (water) and youngest

son (earth) and oldest daughter (wood),
second daughter (fire), and youngest daughter (metal).

In this book, I look at how we can use the model of the bagua to analyze our life, to clear blockages holding us back from where we want to be, and to create harmony and balance in our lives.

How the Book is Organized

When we use Feng Shui in a house, we first clear the clutter and clean the space. Then we cleanse it from any destructive energy and apply a cure with the intention of bringing harmony in the lives of the participants. In the same way, I hope that this book will help you clear clutter—old debilitating emotions and habits— from your life. As you cleanse your life, I will help you come up with cures that will enhance your path to mastery.

The first chapter looks at your journey or path through life. This area relates to your career but, more than that, how well you are in touch with your purpose and how you are flowing through life.

The second chapter looks at your relationships with friends, family, spouse or significant other. This area of the bagua deals with partnerships and close associations, whether these are through marriage. family, friendship or business.

The third chapter looks at your relationship with your parents or elders. This section probes your relationship as to what came before you, your ancestors, and the history or roots that are important to you.

The fourth chapter deals with the area of wealth and blessings. It has to do with the ability to acquire money, as well as the ability to attract blessings and good fortune.

The fifth chapter represents the Tai Chi, the center of the bagua. This area represents health when all other areas are cleared and in harmony.

The sixth chapter deals with the area of helpful people or mentors. We will explore ways of identifying or attracting people who can be helpful to you, as well as ways you can be helpful. These helpers might be people or they may be helpful acts which seem like angels have originated them. This is the area of the bagua that also has to do with travel.

The seventh chapter deals with your creativity and things that you produce. It also includes children. We will look at living with joy and the open expression of creativity, as well as ways of being supportive of your children's growth.

The eighth chapter provides tools for knowing yourself better or looking within. We will examine how much private time we take to really understand ourselves and connect with Spirit.

In the ninth chapter, we explore ways to become known for the person that we are to others, not in the worldly sense of being famous, but in the sense of being a light and inspiration to others.

The chapter numbers that I have chosen also correspond with the numbers which are given to these areas of the bagua. Each one has a trigram and element related to it. I will introduce each chapter by explaining the trigram's meaning. There are eight trigrams and the T'ai Chi at the center. As we look at issues that arise for all of us and cause us blocks, I will tell you about obstacles that I've encountered in my own life and how I have been helped past the blocks by these Eastern principles and practices and the underlying Taoist philosophy. Hopefully these insights will help you.

Although this book does not explain about the practice of Feng Shui in detail, I give you some Feng Shui suggestions for the bagua area of your house and tell you where it is located. Traditional Feng Shui assigns a compass direction to each trigram. All branches of Feng Shui believe that the intention of the person making changes in their environment is crucial to changing the energy.

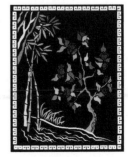

Since I blend Western and Eastern methods, I include psychological practices which will help you solidify your intention to make powerful changes in your life. Most important are the use of affirmations and visualizations. In the next section, I will give you a brief description of both techniques and the underlying theory behind them.

Affirmations and Visualizations

Affirmations or autosuggestions are the suggestions we say to ourselves to change old behavior. Visualizations are the mental pictures that we create to see ourselves differently. Understanding the effect that the mind has on the body, these techniques are extremely important in changing our conditioned thinking.

Before we explain how to use these techniques, it is important to understand what we know of how the subconscious mind works.

WE become what we think about

It appears that the brain and nervous system are influenced by mental images. What we have thought about, from the time we are children, tends to be how we view life. What we have been told by an authority figure, often repeatedly and with a great deal of emotion, tends to stay with us. This is how negative programming takes place. We hear these things so often that they tend to be the lenses through which we view life.

Our thought patterns influence our behavior

Our actions are influenced by the world view that we have about ourselves and the situations around us. If we act in a way that drives people away, it is because we have learned, through our upbringing, that people cannot be trusted and it will hurt to get close to them. On the other hand, if we are open and trusting, we have learned, through caring interactions with people, that some people can be trusted.

The subconscious mind is more powerful than reason

We all do things that we know are not good for us. We realize that what is impressed in the subconscious mind has much more influence than rational ideas. What we have learned about ourselves and our early behavior is so ingrained that, even though we try to change it, we are always drawn back to it. We know that we want to change, but our destructive behavior seems almost out of our control.

The only way to replace a habit is by becoming conscious of it

Our behavior is usually unconscious. We do not even question it, unless it is causing us or someone else harm. The first step is to become conscious of what we are doing. The Eastern practices make us focus inward and become aware of what is happening in our bodies and how our emotional patterns connect to our bodies.

When an idea is accepted, it remains until another one replaces it

The longer we have acted in a certain way, the harder it is to change our behavior. "It is hard to teach an old dog new tricks," the saying goes. However, all behaviors can be changed by replacing limiting thought patterns with new ones. Our thoughts control our behavior. Working on changing our thoughts, through affirmations and visualizations, will produce new behavior.

Each thought creates a physical reaction

Our thoughts influence our bodies by constantly changing the chemical balance. For example, it is well known that constant worry over time will create ulcers. Our body is constantly reacting to the ideas which we are having and, if these thoughts are about worry, doubt, fear, or anger, we are producing the stress response. If we change our thoughts to positive thoughts, we will be sending healthy chemicals through our body. In this book, we work at changing our thoughts.

Each suggestion acted upon creates less opposition to successive suggestions

Through affirmations, you are giving yourself conscious

suggestions which are geared to changing your behavior. You will find that, as you start to act on these suggestions, you will have less resistance to them. Start with simple suggestions and then make them more complicated. As things start to change in your life, as a result of these suggestions, it will be easier to change other behavior.

Rules of Affirmations

Use the present tense

Always give yourself the suggestion as if you are already doing it. For example, Emile Coué, a pioneer in the power of positive thinking, came up with the statement, translated from the French, "Day by day, in every way, I'm getting better and better." This impresses on the subconscious mind the progressive movement toward the state of happiness.

Be positive

Always express what you want to do, not what you do not want to do. Your mind has already been bombarded with negative suggestions so you want to always phrase everything in the way you would like it to happen; for example, " I sleep well all night" instead of "I do not stay awake all night."

Be specific

Choose one specific thing that you want and how you want it. Do not lump together several things that you want as this will confuse the subconscious mind. For example, say to yourself, "I have a perfect relationship in my life" instead of "I have the perfect relationship, I have lost 5 pounds and I sleep all night." Affirm one thing at a time.

Be Detailed

The more detail you use in your autosuggestions or affirmations, the more real they become to the subconscious mind. Use details describing exactly what it will be like when you have what you are affirming; for example, "I am poised, calm and confident as I stand in front of a crowd delivering a speech," instead of "I am an excellent public speaker."

Affirm Activity

Use suggestions that describe action rather than an ability. For example, "I take interest in people around me" rather than "I am a care-giver."

Use emotional and exciting words

Use words such as "vibrant, powerful, exciting, delightful" since the subconscious mind seems to respond more to words that denote feeling.

Be Realistic

Use statements which are in the realm of possibility. I believe that anything is possible but you have to achieve it in small increments. So make your statement about something which you can achieve soon and then you can change these statements as you go along. For example, a statement for someone trying to lose weight would make more sense if the person suggests that she or he is losing 3 pounds a week as opposed to 30 pounds in two months. It is better for the subconscious mind to know that it can achieve results.

Personalize

Make every autosuggestion or affirmation about yourself and your own activity instead of trying to change anyone else. We often try to fashion changes in our children or our spouse but we have no control over them.

Do It With Emotion

The more emotion we use for these suggestions, the more they become impressed in our subconscious mind. As you say the suggestion, really feel yourself having the desired result.

Do It With Activity

As you are making your suggestion, affirm the activity

which would take you to the desired result. For example, say "I am writing three pages a day" instead of "I am a writer."

WRITE IT

When you have an affirmation formulated, write it down so you can look at it. The more senses that you get involved, the more real it becomes to the subconscious mind.

SAY IT OUT LOUD

As you say it out loud, you are also involved in hearing what you want to occur. It is best not to say it with unsupportive people in hearing range because they will often question the validity of what you are doing and start to introduce doubt.

Try to believe that it is possible

Even though the desired result may be far beyond what you have ever had in your life, anything is possible. As you feel that, you will be able to impress your subconscious mind that it is true.

Rules of Visualization

IMAGES

From what we know about impressing the subconscious mind, the more vivid the image that we have about what we are trying to bring into our lives, the more we impress it on this mind and start to produce it in our lives. What we should picture in our mind is the scene of having achieved what we want and make it as real as possible, getting in touch with the joy of being there. Sometimes we think that we know exactly what we want but, when it comes to us, it does not bring the feelings that we want. The better thing is to concentrate on the essence or the feelings that we want to have and picture ourselves having these feelings. You can create the desired feeling before the event happens.

Symbols

From what we know about the mind, it records our experiences in symbols so, in order to communicate with the mind, it is good to picture what you want in symbols. For example, if you are thinking of starting a business, think of something that would symbolize the business to you and get that picture in your mind.

Feel love for your creation

Concentrate on the good feelings you have for what you are visualizing and how good you feel about it. If it is something that can be of service to people, the better you feel about it, the more you will transfer this feeling to people.

Concentration

The more we hold fast to this picture in our mind, the more we become magnetic to what we want.

Remain peaceful

The most important part of this process is that we stay peaceful. If we start to throw doubt into what we are doing, we will hold back the process. This book presents many practices to help you remain peaceful. Once you have decided what you want, you have planted the seed. Know that what you want will manifest so detach from the outcome. This is what the Taoists call non-attachment, described in Chapter 8.

Replace a word with a feeling

In the same way as using a symbol, you can use a word that you can program to bring certain feelings. For example, every time that you think of the word tree, allow yourself to feel peaceful and calm, lying under a tree, with the sun relaxing your body or a gentle breeze on your face.

Use the Time just before you go to sleep and when you wake up

The time that we are most in touch with our subconscious mind, and therefore more suggestible, is just before sleep and when we wake up in the morning. This is a time

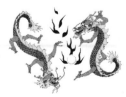

when our visualizations and suggestions will be most accepted.

Make it simple

The most important part of this is to make it easy without effort. The more simple and unforced you make this process of visualizing and affirming, the more profoundly it will work.

Be aware of these powerful tools as you do the exercises at the end of the chapters in this book.

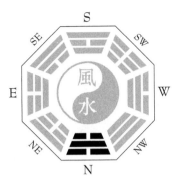

CHAPTER 1
THE JOURNEY

Journey Trigram

The first trigram is one unbroken yang line sandwiched between two broken yin lines. In terms of the archetypal family, it represents the middle son. The Chinese name for this is "K'an" and it means deep water. In this deep water, we plumb our depths for meaning in our life. In some sense this area represents our career, but it is more than that. This is our path or journey through life—the way we steer our course. As in good Feng Shui, when we proceed step by step, more mystery is revealed to us.

Here is the area where we search our purpose or destiny. Because of the element of water, the ebb and flow of life is underscored. The colors represented here are black or a deep blue, like the depths of the ocean. It is on the North side of your house.

In the bagua, the journey trigram is opposite the trigram for fame or reputation and the two are closely related. It is the way you take your journey through life that allows you to become the person for whom you are known. In this chapter, we will look at embarking on our journey, being in the flow, finding

1

purpose in our life, dealing with change and seeing life as a circle.

Embarking

For any journey, we must embark. When we go on a trip, we leave to go somewhere and we come back at a later date. Our experiences have changed us into a different person.

Our journey through life is much the same. We go from experience to experience and each one changes us. We interpret some as bad and some as good. Each one has its impact and gives us another way of seeing things.

If we look at life as a school, we are investing in an education, increasing our knowledge as we go along. Some of these courses seem more difficult than others, but they all help us to grow and evolve.

As we embark on this journey towards knowing ourselves better, we look at what we have learned so far and assess its meaning in order to continue with new awareness. What we sense is that this is a special path we are now on with new rules and understanding. We may not know exactly how it is different, but we feel that it is.

An important first step is to assess all parts of our lives in order to move forward on our journey because this is a crucial time for our personal transformation. The metaphysical texts of all cultures point to the present time for a shift in consciousness. It does not matter what you have come through to get to this point. It only matters how you proceed from now on.

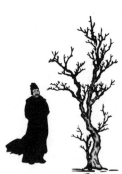

You may have been in places where you didn't want to be psychologically, emotionally or financially, and you may still be stuck in those places. You do not have to remain there. You can get unstuck and move through those blocks to a more joyous, abundant life. We are all in the process of moving forward all the time.

Let's look at the element of water.

Consider the movement of water and see how it flows from place to place. If you have ever watched the flowing of a stream, you will see that it is hard to contain water in one place. It continues to flow. It may have obstacles on the path, boulders and dams, but it finds its way around them. Water can be very gentle but persistent and wears down anything in its path.

Continuing with the metaphor of water, sometimes it is like a torrent and other times it is like a little trickle and sometimes it has hardly any movement, as in the winter when it is under ice. Just know that water has the potential of a tidal wave.

You have the same potential. Your life might be operating at the level of a trickle now or you may be quiescent, waiting for something to get you moving again. Just know that whatever stage you are at, things will change. If they are moving at hurricane force, there will be a time when they will slow down. Each stage is there for a reason.

When I left Canada to come to the United States, it was a time for me when things appeared to be out of control. For some reason, my whole life was disrupted. I disagreed with the autocratic leadership of a new dean in my department at the university. Threatened by this disagreement, or, in his words, insubordination, he fired me from my administrative job, even though I continued to teach in another section of the university.

At the same time, I lost money in a land deal, my ex-husband stopped supporting my children, and my other business was not doing well. The pressure of all these things was causing difficulty in my relationship with my partner at that time, now my present husband. These challenges forced me to take stock of my life and to move forward in another direction. I ended up in Florida doing my present work. If these things had not happened to me, I might have become stuck and refused to move on, but I had no choice.

Sometimes we get caught up in our experiences and, just like Odysseus in the Odyssey, get stuck in certain places and don't want to continue. Either these places feel good or we don't know how to extract ourselves. If we look at all our experiences as either boulders that hold us back or as a straight pathway that moves our stream along, we can evaluate our lives from a perspective that makes the journey easier. The main thing to remember is that sometimes, to get into the flow of life, we need to crash past boulders that seem almost impossible to circumvent. When I look back now at my life at that time, if I hadn't been forced to deal with the obstacles, I might have allowed them to stay in my path. If I had concentrated on what appeared to be insurmountable difficulties, I might not have found the strength to move forward. Instead I discovered, as I moved with the stream of life, that there seemed to be something bigger than me supporting me on my path.

To put this in a spiritual perspective, imagine that you are a drop of water in the ocean. You have all the characteristics of the ocean, you contain everything that the ocean contains, but you are only a small part of it. This is the part that we play in the universal scheme of things. We have all the characteristics of the whole universe, but we are only a small part of it. The universe does not exist outside us. We are as much a part of it as a drop of ocean water is part of the ocean and we need our connection to the universe as much as the drop of ocean water needs the ocean. We cannot exist apart from it as much as we might try.

I like to imagine myself as a stream destined to become part of a large body of water. This is our path, as earthly wanderers, to find that destination and become part of a larger body of water. If I had not had that adversity, I might not have searched

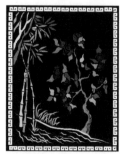 for more spirituality in my life. Our earthly experiences are all geared towards helping us, as drops of water, move along the path towards joining with the ocean. As much as we get caught up with other things, just remember that the main goal of life is to work around the obstacles and stay in the flow.

Staying in the Flow

One of the major differences between the Western view and the view of Taoism is that, in the West, we live in the future. We set goals to which we strive and, oftentimes, are concentrating more on the future than the present. Our minds are whirling with thoughts of the past or future and we rarely concentrate on the present.

How many times have you gone somewhere in your car and not remembered how you got there? We are often so preoccupied that we are not aware of what is around us. Being in the flow is the Taoist way of living in the moment, not in the future. How do we justify living in the flow when we are told that we are to set goals and have specific plans for our life?

The *Tao Te Ching* tells us that "a good traveler has no fixed plans." This reminds us that we should make our decisions and choices not by schedule but according to the information we receive intuitively from moment to moment. Living in the flow means trusting the universe to send you messages and following them to create your path. An image to hold in mind is moving along smoothly with the current in a boat without bothering to steer it because you are open to wherever it takes you.

How do we reconcile this with goal setting? It is true that people who set goals have more control over what happens in their lives. It is also important to know that there might be an even better plan for your life and, if you are trying to force yourself to get there in a certain way, you may be moving against your ultimate purpose. There are also many people who have very specific goals that they want to meet and they move towards those goals against all obstacles and find that is not where they wanted to be in the first place. They got the job or the lifestyle of their dreams only to find that it was an empty illusion.

I have many clients who have good professions and are earning excellent salaries but they are not happy. From the time that they were children they were told that they should strive to be in their chosen profession. They do as they are told but find that there is something lacking. They were concentrating on that goal and often turned away from things that were presented to them at the time. Now, as they look back, they wish they had taken another course. They know that they have missed out on other opportunities that would have made them happier.

On the other hand, there are people who sit and do nothing waiting for things to happen and they wile away their lives creating nothing. What we need to achieve is the happy balance between these two—allowing ourselves to connect with the feelings of the moment, as well have some kind of goals for our life. How do we do this?

I believe the key is that we have an idea about where we want to go but we don't know how we are going to get there. It is important to know the feeling that you want to have once you have achieved your goal but not to be rigidly attached to how you are going to achieve it.

If we do indeed have a higher purpose or there is a divine plan for our lives, how do we connect with it? This is where we use Eastern practices to slow down our minds and help us to recognize the clues around us. We are always being sent messages from the universe, whether it be events which happen around us or people who come into our life at certain times. These clues may come in words we read or hear someone say at just the right moment.

How can we live this on a daily basis, always searching for the synchronicity of situations and not get caught up in the drama around us? We must know when to move and when to stay still and listen. Even when everything is rushing around you, be able to go into yourself and check in with your feelings. Your innermost feelings will let you know whether what you are doing feels good or not. By checking with your feelings, you are connecting with the intuition and guidance which is your connection to your higher self, the part of you which has all the answers for your life from a higher perspective.

These answers, I believe, can be found by calmly focusing on the present, but we are so afraid of staying still and doing nothing. Our culture has taught us, from the time we were children, to always be active and plan for the future. We teach children to run around wildly, running from activity to activity, not knowing that they have a choice to do anything else. .

To be in the present is really the only place we can be, even though we think otherwise. How many times have you sat in the stillness of nature and let everything go from your mind? What if you took one day off and just sat, being aware of only what was going on in the present?

If you have done this before, you know that, once you drop the anxiety of not getting things done, you will start to notice things that you have never seen before. Maybe you have never noticed the color and texture of the things around you.

As you sit, you will start to get inner urges or intuitive understandings about certain things or events in your life. If you follow through on these hunches, you might meet someone who will introduce you to something which might change your life. You might follow an urge to write or paint or create something which, in the end, will change your career. Living in the present will help you connect with your purpose.

Finding Purpose

As we live in the present and stay open to synchronicity in situations and clues from the universe, we will start to see that there appears to be a certain way we are to live our life. That is our purpose. How do we know that we are on the right path towards the expression of that purpose? I have learned that it takes trial and error before we really find the smooth way. Even then, what appears to be the wrong path helps us to understand the process of life better.

In my own life, the abrupt transition taking me away from secure work out into the world, not being sure what I was going to do, felt like failure at the time. Looking from my perspective today, I needed that period of uncertainty and instability to take stock and really think about what I wanted to do.

I learned that life is not usually straightforward and we try many paths before we get one that feels like it fits. In fact, it may be necessary to go on many paths before we find the one that flows smoothly and I believe that this is part of the process. Finding purpose has to do with how we spend our time each day, and how we influence or impact the world. For some of us, it has nothing to do with career, but for most of us our career path has a great deal to do with it. When I lost my job, I started to think about the things that I liked to do on a daily basis and realized that these pursuits, like studying Eastern philosophy, doing Eastern practices, and teaching and counseling people could be combined into a career. However, I realized also that all the things that I had done in the past had given me important experiences and could be incorporated into what I am doing today.

Like many people, I found my path through a very circuitous route. After graduating from university, I had decided that I did not want to do what everyone was doing which was to teach high school. I ended up working for an insurance company and finding work that was interesting, but not engrossing. I paid claims and there were many people who were making disability claims for all types of problems. Much to the company's dismay, I got involved in people's problems and became their champion as to why the claim should be paid. It was then that I began to realize that my real interest was in people and their problems. Also I was seeing that, in many of our systems, people were viewed as statistics instead of individuals with challenges in their lives. I left this business when I became pregnant with my first child.

When my children were growing up, I did a lot of volunteer work with different groups and found that I focused on work with people. I got particularly involved in the Distress Center, helping people on the phone with their problems. It was then I knew that there were a lot of lonely and desperate people because this service provided a lifeline, especially for people who were suicidal. I started thinking about how people's think-ing patterns can influence their lives so negatively. People con-templating suicide felt that they had no recourse and that this was the only way out. Even with my limited knowledge at the time I worked with them, trying to help them to let go of debil-itating thinking patterns, and to look at other options, finding hope instead of devastation. Over the years, it has underscored for me the importance of the basic teaching of the Feng Shui bagua, to let go of old blockages in order to balance all areas of your life.

My next volunteer work was with people of many different cultures, including Native Indians, West Indians, Asians and Europeans found living in Toronto, Canada at the time. I became aware that people had so many ways of looking at the same thing, each influenced by the cultural filter through which they viewed it. What became apparent was that so many people think that their way of seeing something is the only one and strike out at people who see things differently. In response to racial violence, perpetuated by that kind of thinking, the com-mittee that I worked for had been set up, in the city of Toronto, to help people understand and be tolerant of other cultures. Racism and bigotry are also thought patterns and, in this vol-unteer work, I helped people understand their own prejudices.

The experience in this volunteer work took me back to graduate school where I studied a combination of counseling and multiracial studies, which eventually led me to my work with Chinese students. Even though I was headed on a path of working with people, and especially those of other cultures, I still worked at other things. I had a clothing store because of my love of fashion and, through my store, got very involved in a multilevel marketing skin care company. At the same time, I was doing administration and counseling and teaching at a uni-versity. My hope, in doing all these things, was to make enough money to be able to be free and on my own. The end result of this is that I ended up chasing so many things at once that all of them suffered and I needed to take on even more work to pay for all the businesses in which I was involved.

I learned from these experiences that doing things for money sometimes takes you away from your purpose. The path that we are seeking is our own niche in the world and, if we look only for money, we will be hard pressed to find this unique place. We often do things that are truly not our passion and compromise ourselves with the justification that when money comes, we will really do what we want to do. We push very hard at something that is not aligned to our purpose and find that the money, even if it comes, is not satisfying us at any deep level.

I have seen many people who have finally succeeded at what they thought they wanted to do and the money is finally there, but they still feel dissatisfied. Studies have verified that emotional problems in older people are related to regrets at not doing things presented to them in their earlier years. I believe that we all have our unique purpose but some of us get lost on the way. Our humanness makes it very difficult to remember why we are here. We get feelings occasionally, inklings and intuitions, which urge us along in certain ways, but often we are too busy to heed them.

Our purpose, then, is to find our unique path in life. How do we know when we are on it? It is when we move with alignment with our passion. It is when we get up every day and love what we are doing. It is moving with synchronicity and inner urges and finding that things seem to flow. When we seem to 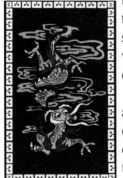 be pushing too hard and things do not flow, then we are working against our purpose. We spend a great deal of our time at work and, if we do not enjoy what we are doing, it destroys our hope for happiness.

When I ask my clients in therapy if they are really doing what they want to do, they often reply that they are not, but they have to do it to make money. I sympathize with this thinking because, as I have just described, I have done this myself. What we need to develop is a way of thinking which affirms that we can do anything we want to do, then let go of fear and believe that money will come from these things. My hope is that, as you complete this circle of the bagua, you will be able to clear away some of the old thinking habits and conditioning that stop you from being truly on the path of your heart.

This part of the bagua is your career, but also your journey through life. What we are looking for is a smooth path that, as we said before, flows like water, moving around and over obstacles but forever moving forward towards our final destination which, as we said, is the destination of enlightenment or really knowing your soul's purpose. As we move forward, let us always be aware that life means forever adapting to change.

Change

In order to clear away the blockages in all areas of our lives, we need to be aware that life is always changing, just as water has a constant ebb and flow.

The *I Ching*, known as the Book of Changes, was formed from combining the eight trigrams in all possible ways, making 64 hexagrams. The meaning of these hexagrams became the basis for ancient teachings which remind us that life is always in a state of flux. The ancient Chinese saw the cosmos as a constant interaction of two forces, Yin and Yang, each carrying the seed of the other.

Two main arms of Chinese philosophy, Taoism and Confucianism, influenced by the *I Ching*, teach us to find the "middle way" which means to seek harmony in the inevitability of this change. Be prepared to make the necessary shifts in your life, at any given moment in order to come back to a balanced and harmonious state.

This reminds me of when I learned about "cognitive dissonance," a psychological theory that says that if you have something that is occurring in your life which does not make sense to your existing belief system, you will either change the situation to be more in harmony with your beliefs or you will change your beliefs. Your mind will naturally seek homeostasis or balance. In this Eastern approach, the balance we seek is in the present moment, based on the information that we have.

This means that, at any given time, you can make immediate decisions about which way to go and what to do. In modern psychological terms, we tend, in the West, to make decisions from pure logic and a rational decision making process. In contrast, when we are guided by intuition and inner knowing, we learn to be more open to our surroundings and the information presented to us in the now.

The *I Ching* assumes that the world as we see it is a reflection of an underlying reality, that all things are connected and are in the process of continuous transformation. According to Taoist, Buddhist, and Confucian thought, the Cosmos is continually in motion, every particle shifting in relation to all others, synchronized in time and space with no time but the present. Carl Jung, who had studied the *I Ching* extensively, came up with the concept of synchronicity, which means "meaningful coincidences" when we get inklings of this underlying reality or messages from the universe.

In the West, our usual concept of time is that it is linear and that it is a straight line which goes from the past to the present. The Eastern approach views time as circular with the past and future always in a state of interaction. The influences of the past have created the present situation which has the seeds of the unfolding of events in the future.

What does that mean to us? It means that change is inevitable and that we can handle life more easily living in the present. We often try to keep things the way they are. As a result, we stop ourselves from moving forward in our lives and miss the opportunities that could be there if we were willing to be open to change.

We get accustomed to things the way they are and try to hold onto them. This holding on creates blockages in our lives. In the same way, if we suppress emotions, we create blockages in our bodies. If we hold onto clutter, we create blockages in our environment.

It is time to be willing to move with change, even though you may not know exactly where it will take you but trusting that you will be able to handle anything that comes up. It is when we get stuck or attached to an outcome of a situation that we become disappointed or disillusioned. If we remain open, we accept whatever appears as appropriate for the situation and move forward with the flow of life.

When we are allowing for change, we are letting life happen. We are taking actions without being attached to the results. We know that there is something beyond our understanding and we realize that we do not know the bigger picture.

We learn that we cannot judge a situation because we do not know the underlying reality, so we move with situations as they happen. When we handle situations like that, we are open to any outcome and we accept the fact that we may not understand the significance until much later on.

I'm sure that you have had things happen which seemed to have an immediate disastrous consequence but, later on, you realized that you would not have developed some positive understanding in your life if it had not been for that event. When my life changed as a result of losing my job, my money, and relationship at the same time, it felt like the end of the world. My understanding was not as it is now and I thought that I had lost everything. As I look back now, the events at this time were the catalyst to move me to a new level of understanding. I was not able to rely on my worldly understanding so I was driven to spiritual books to open myself up to a power beyond this world. When I began to espouse these principles, I stopped resisting change and instead started to welcome it. Starting to flow with life and watching for synchronicity in situations, through a flow of events that I will describe elsewhere, I moved to another location and was drawn to my present work.

When things happen to you, whether it be a breakup of a

relationship, a failure in business, an accident, the loss of a job etc., know that things are not as they seem. As horrible as it appears at the time, you will see that, later on, this event has moved you to a new perspective on life. As you look back, you will be thankful for the experience.

Know that, as you progress on your journey, many things will come your way. Try not to judge them. Just be open to the experience, knowing that you can never take a wrong turn. Because everything in life is circular, you can never be off the path.

Life is a Circle

As we embark on this journey of life, we become aware of symbols that have a deeper meaning. In Feng Shui, symbols are important. It is believed that they have an impact on us consciously and subconsciously. Subconsciously, we create the symbols in our environment. If we use the symbol of a circle for our life and think of our journey as circular, then where we start, we end up; what we send out, we get back.

A circle is unending, its resistance is minimal. Look at the symbol of the T'ai Chi. The symbol represents the combination of opposite energies, Yin and Yang. These energies, just as in the symbol, flow into one another and each contains the seed of the other. Yin represents qualities such as stillness, yielding, closing, softness, and insubstantial, while Yang represents qualities such as movement, opening, hardness, action, and substantial. Even these processes are circular because they flow into each other and each can't exist without the opposite part.

Our life is a combination of these energies, and often one is labeled bad and the other good, but one cannot exist without the other. We cannot have dark without light, love without hate, beauty without ugliness. How do we know what love is until we have experienced hate or know what light is without darkness? Neither is bad or good. One is just the absence of the other, but they are interconnected and need each other to exist in our world. We often spend a great deal of energy resisting the experience or situation or people that we label as bad. However, to balance the polarities in our life, the key is to embrace them rather than resist them.

As our perception changes and we see that everything has a right to exist, we start to release the things that no longer serve us and move away from situations that no longer blend with our energy. If we look at nature, we get good examples of how that happens. Water in a stream does not accuse a rock of being in its path. It does not say "I hate you and must obliterate you" but, instead, flows around it. It does not fear the rock, but finds a way around it.

Let us look at our own lives and see what we are resisting. If we remember that life is a circle, we will remember again that what we are putting out will come back to us. When we resist certain situations, we find that life presents these situations to us over and over again. Again, we remember that what we resist persists. We need to look at the negative qualities of our lives and see them differently. Are the things which we judge as negative just showing us the opposite quality? We have to learn to flow between these states - moving from negative to positive, active to passive, strong to weak.

Sometimes it is appropriate in our lives to pull back and other times it is better to move forward and be active. No state is any better or worse than another—there is a time and place for both. If we look at life in terms of the elements, there is a time to prepare under the surface (water), a time to go forward (wood), a time to move at our highest energy (fire), a time to pull back (metal) and a time for stillness (earth). I know now that what appeared to be a very weak time of my life, when I had lost everything, was a time of preparation in which I began to look more seriously at the *Tao Te Ching* and other Eastern philosophy as well as spiritual literature. I became open to new opportunities and found myself in South Florida doing workshops. It was time to seize the moment and go forward. If I had not had that time of introspection, I

15

would not have been ready to move. What appeared to be a difficult situation ended up moving me onto my chosen path in life.

In the scheme of things, there is a place for crime, for so-called evil and every other experience. In fact, I believe that there is no accident on earth, that these situations exist to show us certain lessons. The esoteric literature reminds us that we live out the wheel of karma, from lifetime to lifetime. Through reincarnation, we complete situations from other lifetimes. Things are never as they seem because we do not have all the information.

As we advance on our path, let us look at all the events and circumstances that remain hidden in our lives. Be aware that everything is circular. Our paths are concentric and, in the end, they all lead to the same place, back to the Source. It does not matter where you are on the path at this time because you can change direction any time. We are all heading to the same place. Some of our lessons take longer to learn than others, but each gives the same message—that we can learn from experience and go on. As we move forward on the journey of life, let us look at the blocks and obstacles that keep us stuck and learn to flow around and over them. The next exercise will help you connect with the path of your heart, which will make your journey smoother.

FiNdiNq PuRpOSE ExERCiSE

How would you spend your day if you could do anything that you wanted to do? List five things that you love to do.

1.

2.

3.

4.

5.

List five qualities that are special about you.

1.

2.

3.

4.

5.

If you were living in a perfect world, what would it be like? What is your vision of the world?

How can you use your special qualities doing the things you like to do to create your perfect world? Doing these things in your unique way can create an impact on the world. This is your purpose and, if you visualize yourself doing these things every day, you will find a way that brings money to you.

Affirmations

I am truly on the path of my heart.

I spend every day doing what I love to do.

I enjoy the present moment.

I move over obstacles on my path with ease.

Feng Shui for Your Environment

This is your journey, your path represented by the element of water. Suggestions for this part of your house are:

- Water fountain or aquarium
- Pictures of water scenes
- Colors of black or dark blue
- Anything representing your career path
- Wavy or amorphous shaped items
- Mirror or glass

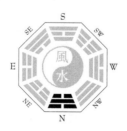

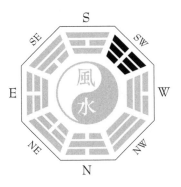

CHAPTER 2
Relationships

Relationship Trigram

The relationship trigram is represented by three broken lines. The Chinese name for this trigram is "K'un" and this, the most yin of all trigrams, is the archetype of the maternal female or the mother. It is the element of earth and the meaning of this trigram is receptive earth. The colors here are earth colors and the color of pink. This is the part of your home that is the most receptive, and the qualities to be emphasized here are yielding, openness and trust. This is the Southwest corner of your house.

In your home and in your life, this is the place to clear away all blocks keeping you from harmonious relationships, particularly intimate relationships and partnerships. In the bagua, it is across from inner knowledge. To be able to give yourself fully in a relationship, you need to be aware of your own limitations and strengths.

In this chapter, we will look at how our own dysfunctional patterns make it hard to have healthy relationships and how a willingness to change them can build happy, fulfilling, harmonious relationships.

Patterns in Relationships

Some of the greatest challenges in our lives come from relationships—whether they are intimate relationships, family relationships or work relationships. Of all the problems which bring people to me as a therapist, relationships appear to cause the most distress. Why is that?

All our insecurities come up full force in our relationships. The situations that hold the seeds of those insecurities, which form our early conditioning, are usually those experienced, with great impact, in the first five years. Frightening, isn't it? Most of our behavior has been learned that early and then reinforced over the years. The things that are ground in the most strongly are the emotionally charged messages that we heard repeatedly from authority figures.

These were often the statements by well-meaning parents who were insecure themselves and did not realize the harm that they were causing. Often they programmed us to believe that we were not good enough or smart enough or our behavior was wrong, no matter what it was. Even worse, some of us were abused in very degrading ways.

Most of us have been brought up with conditional love; that is, we feel that we are loved more when we act one way as opposed to another. We start to behave in the way that gets approval and submerge our own desires and feelings. These repressed feelings cause us to develop patterns of behavior that are dysfunctional. There are several patterns, very predominant in relating to others, that I have observed.

I AM NOT WORTHY

Since, in some cases, we feel that our parents did not value us, we learn not to value ourselves. We show this pattern by not accepting anything good for ourselves and not thinking we deserve anything, especially a good relationship. Unconsciously, people in this pattern attract to themselves similar partners who project their own disapproval of themselves back onto them. It is in the intimacy of a relationship that we repeat our early childhood patterns and reveal our insecurity or even self-hate.

There is often a fear of abandonment because, as children, a parent often abandoned us, either physically or emotionally. This fear is usually realized because unconsciously we act in a way to end the relationship or the relationship continues in an abusive manner.

When this pattern becomes extreme, it can turn into violence in a relationship. A violent man (or woman) is filled with self-loathing and projects that onto his partner. His brutal attempt to control the relationship shows his desperate fear of being abandoned. He has usually witnessed or has been a victim of violence in his own home.

This feeling of unworthiness keeps us in relationships where often we are not honored. It is when we start to honor ourselves that the dynamic of the relationship starts to change.

You owe me something

This pattern emerges with people who have not received the love and affection that they craved in their early childhood, so they spend their lives searching for it. These people are very demanding and, no matter what you give them, it is not enough, because that inner desire is not satisfied. They always complain about what they haven't received and feel that they have not been given what they are owed.

When we feel this way, we become dissatisfied with relationships and we are always waiting for the other person to do something for us. As we begin to give ourselves the love and attention that we are missing, then we can stop relying on someone else to do it.

You complete me

This is more apt to be prevalent in an intimate relationship when someone loses his or her identity in a relationship. This pattern emerges when a child has not been allowed to develop his or her own power. Also it develops when we search for a feeling of complete happiness, like a time in our early childhood when we had the unwavering attention and affection of a caregiver. Conversely we may never have received this feeling and, therefore, we crave it.

When we first become involved in an intimate relationship, we give ourselves entirely to the other person, trying to fill their every need, giving selflessly. Often the other person does the same and we feel completed in every aspect. This can turn into a co-dependent relationship in which both partners try to complete themselves through the other, never standing strong on their own. This becomes very unhealthy because we focus our attention on our partner instead of ourselves. We try to act in a way that satisfies the expectations of our partner and get upset if our partner doesn't do the same. Usually this pattern continues until one of the members decides to concentrate on himself/herself. With this shift in the existing dysfunctional pattern, the other partner starts to blame and feels bitter. The only way of moving through this pattern is to find our own power and stand securely on our own.

YOU ARE OUT TO GET ME

I have seen this pattern manifest itself in families at the time of a parent's death when members of a family get involved in squabbles over a will. This divisiveness was encouraged early in children's lives. Parents, brought up in a similar manner, would encourage competition and backstabbing. Often money and possessions took precedence over love and caring in these families.

Sometimes this infighting doesn't even have to be about money. The fight can occur over some family principle which ends up with members of the family not talking to one another for years. I see people who have all their energy completely embroiled in these kinds of family battles.

In intimate relationships, this pattern shows up in the feeling that your partner is taking advantage of you, leaving you feeling suspicious and mistrusting. When we are so tied up with this kind of thinking, we are totally out of our own power. We become so obsessed with others' behavior that eventually we can even get sick. I have known people to ruminate about the treatment they have received from others to such an extent that they can't enjoy life fully. As we start to develop a sense of ourselves as strong spiritual beings, we will start to realize that nothing or nobody on the outside can influence us.

I AM A VICTIM

There are many people who feel that they have no control over their lives. This pattern begins developing in children who see powerlessness modeled by parents and society. For example, in relationships where a child who has had at least one domineering parent or has seen one parent dominated by the other tends to develop this pattern. In this case, the child models either the dominant or the submissive parent. As I mentioned before, both patterns usually come from a feeling of not being worthy.

The feeling of victimization leaves us feeling powerless in our lives. For women, this feeling is especially prevalent since, in many homes, the male is dominant and makes all the decisions. Children learn that they are simply victims of circumstances and that they have to submit to the expectations of others.

This pattern often manifests in women who, later on, get into situations where husbands abuse them. Subconsciously we attract situations which prove to us, over and over again, that we are victims. This pattern continues until we realize that we do have our own power and do not need to be victims.

Purpose of Relationships

The purpose of relationships in our lives is to reveal to us our patterns so we can work through them and heal them. Some people would prefer to remove themselves from relationships rather than deal with the challenges that relationships give them. I often find people who have given up on intimate relationships, and they tell me that they are so much more peaceful on their own. People who have made this decision usually exhibit some bitterness against old relationships. What they don't look at is the gift of self-knowledge given to them by a difficult relationship. When people tell me that they are more content alone, I remind them that, to truly know themselves, they have to find the patterns that keep them from being peaceful in a relationship.

We attract to ourselves people who are a mirror of our dysfunction. The parts of the other people, which we dislike the most, are often hidden parts of ourselves. For example, in my own life, my first marriage was to a man who held onto anger as I did.

We had very little communication and eventually ended up getting divorced.

My second husband helped me to face my own repressed anger. When he would fight with me and show me his rage, I eventually started to fight back and found that I, too, was dealing with the same emotions. I had expectations of this man that he was not fulfilling and I was angry and resentful. I was also sick of his explosive way of handling things. My father handled things in much the same way and I had spent my early life trying either to pacify his anger or not pro-voke it. Expressing my own anger was a new behavior for me, since it was not allowed in my home, and I realized later that I was releas-ing years of repressed feelings.

I left this husband for a period of time because of our continuous fighting, thinking that there was no solution for our relationship except separation. But when I left, things changed. At first, there was a lot of bitterness but, as we got used to the idea that we were apart, we both started to understand our own patterns, began to strengthen ourselves spiritually and find our own power. More importantly, we let go of our expectations of one another. When we met with the intention of doing the final legal separation, we found that, with the old expectations gone, we got along much better. One of the hardest behaviors to give up is our expectation of others.

Expectations of Others

We learn, as small children, to do what others expect of us. In fact, we are rewarded or punished according to how well we carry out the expectations of others. We learn to get praise from our parents or early caregivers by doing approved things. After a while, we start to behave in a way that will please others or, if we choose to be rebel-lious, in a way that will upset others. Both behaviors are meant to get a reaction and, as we grow, we get more and more out of touch with what will please us.

We are taught that concentrating on pleasing ourselves is selfish, that we must take everyone else into consideration before ourselves. The problem is that we begin to know ourselves not as individual beings but only in relation to others. We do not know where we end

and others begin, nor understand what psychologists call the boundary between who we are and who others are. When we are young,
this often makes us feel like we are part of a tight family system.
Children who are not part of a structure end up feeling like they don't
belong anywhere and often develop emotional problems. On the
other hand, children who have no sense of themselves can also end
up emotionally disturbed. These children learn not to trust their own
instincts.

As adults, we are often caught between doing what we want to do
and what others want us to do. In our jobs, we must follow the con-
fines of other peoples' expectations for many hours a day. If we live
in a family, we must accommodate to the wishes of a spouse or parent
or even our children. Often we are left with feelings of frustration of
having to carry out certain obligations every day. As a therapist, I see
many people who are not living their own lives at all — only other
people's expectations.

As I mentioned before, in studies looking at older people who had
severe health problems and even mental illness, we see repeatedly the
theme of not having lived their own lives. They regretted not doing
things that had been presented to them earlier and it was now too
late. They were filled with remorse and regret for having lived for
other people, not themselves.

How do we live our lives for ourselves, not others? It is only in
the North American and some other Western cultures that we have
the luxury of this choice. In many cultures throughout the world,
rigid codes must be adhered to. For Easterners, strict family values
are built into their culture and there is a sense of collective community. This structure can enhance the community but can put great
pressure on the individual. We will look at the value of these communities, however, in another chapter.

For now let us look at how living according to the expectations of
others can hold us back. I was brought up to value my parents' opinion on everything. They were very judgmental on most subjects and
I learned their way of looking at things. They had valuable opinions
and were open minded on many things but very close-minded on
others.

As I left home to go to university at 18 years of age, I realized that many of their views did not apply to my new life. However, I was plagued by a feeling of guilt for not doing what others wanted me to do. My father used to tell me, over and over again, that I was selfish or that I was headstrong and that I did what I wanted to do instead of what he wanted me to do. The overall feeling that it left me with was not to value my own feelings and that everything that I did was wrong. He would say repeatedly that I only thought of myself and not of others.

This has played out in my later years as the old feeling of guilt that comes up whenever I feel that I have not done what others want me to do. For example, I often have this feeling when people want me to work with them or do things for them even though I know that I don't want to do it. As you know in your own life, there are always people wanting you to do something. You have to be very vigilant in every situation to know what is someone else's wish of you and what is your own.

It is easy to get caught up with the emotion of guilt and acquiesce to others' expectations or remain feeling guilty because you did not. When that feeling surfaces around a relationship, I stop and acknowledge that it has more to do with the past than the present.

Those of us who do too much for others become martyrs and eventually resent people. We may even feel guilty because we feel this resentment. What we need is that sense of balance between our desires and the desires of others. When we do things for other people, we need to do it from our heart. We need to feel our own power before we can give to others. We cannot give to anyone from an empty well.

We have all been in relationships when others have become resentful and blaming and we know instinctively that it has nothing to do with us. We may feel somewhat to blame, but that is because we are reacting from old behavior. Our parents may have felt overwhelmed with other problems and felt burdened by us. Indirectly or directly, they may have made us feel that we were to blame for everything. When this feeling comes upon us, in later relationships, we are reenacting the old situation and we need to stand back and become aware of it.

When we start to take care of ourselves and really honor our own desires and needs, we start to feel complete and whole. More importantly, we need to respect ourselves as spiritual beings. We need spiritual sustenance to really feel whole, but that means finding our own way of dealing with spirit. There are many religious institutions that also put huge expectations on their followers, leaving them feeling very guilty.

Our main objective, then, is to find a way that we can live without shame and guilt, honoring our own path. When you start to feel guilt in dealing with others or in doing something displeasing to another, take a good look at the situation. Is this your wish or is it another's? To really be true to yourself, to honor your spirit and your purpose here on earth, you need to do what is right for you—even if it disappoints another. In the same way, we have to give up our need to control others.

Giving Up Control

As well as having things expected of us, we also develop expectations of others. One of the hardest things to give up in relationships is our own need for control. We have an image of how we want our relationship to work and we try to manipulate our own as well as other people's behavior to fit this mold. The problem is that we can only control our own behavior, not anybody else's. Also, that rigid way of trying to get something to fit into place takes us away from another possible way the relationship can unfold.

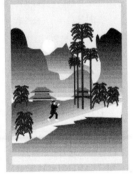

We develop this need for control from our early upbringing. In order to socialize us into society, our parents or early caregivers controlled what we did, where we went and even what we should think. As we get older, we hope that our parents will teach us to think on our own, make our own decisions and take control of our own lives. Usually, however, parents continue to expect us to stay within the value system and the structure that they have taught us.

In many cases, we eventually rebel against our parents' authority and start to live our lives according to a structure contrary to our parents' values. Usually we have not examined our own values or how we want to live life. We move blindly into a career or a relationship and start to adapt to the structure and controls set by the work environment or the other person in our relationship.

That is why, often in middle age, we stop and rebel against our lives, in what is known as the mid-life crisis. We wake up one morning and find that we are carrying out our lives according to rote. "What do we really want?" we ask. Are we living what we want or according to someone else's plan? At this time, when we get in touch with who we are and what we want, we often revise our life and go in another direction or continue the same way with a little more consciousness.

Another scenario is one in which we have been brought up with no controls at all by parents who were completely inconsistent and we search for that structure through a rigid religious institution or even something as inflexible as a gang or a cult. It is our inherent need for some kind of structure which leads us to these confining situations.

It is also this need which drives us to want to control people in our relationships. We think that we know the best way to proceed and we try to merge other people's wishes with our own. We become controlling as lovers, spouses, friends and even parents. Our deep-seated insecurity makes us feel better if we can regulate other people.

Taken to the extreme, one person (usually a man) tries to control a partner's comings and goings and becomes violent if the other person tries to do something for herself. There are too many examples of women maimed or killed by old lovers or husbands when they tried to leave a controlling, abusive situation.

I have had many friends, acquaintances and business colleagues who try to control me. Perhaps it is my non-argumentative nature that attracts them to me. Because I had controlling parents, I try often to accommodate to their wishes until I realize that I am doing things against my instincts. I have become involved in many major investments that were completely in the control of others to the point that I lost a great deal of money.

I have also had my day of trying to control other people in relationships, thinking that I knew the better way for things to be done. After all, there has to be a leader, one person who shows the other the best way. I realize, after a broken marriage and children who have been rebellious at different times, that I had to relinquish control. This is difficult because I have one of my adult children still living with me. When I see him doing things that alarm me, I would like to change the situation but I know that I cannot. At this point, it is up to him to find his own path and learn his own lessons in his own way.

How do we do that? We need to trust that there is a divine plan and that we all have different roles to play in this world and that we cannot possibly know what the other person is supposed to do. In any relationship, it is best to let go and support that person in what he or she wants to do, even if we do not agree with it.

We have to let go of the relationship as well. The paradox is that the more we hold on to a relationship, the more pressure we put on it. If we develop ourselves to the point that we feel complete within ourselves and we know that we do not rely on another, we are then capable of having a truly good relationship. It is a Taoist principle that to be truly strong, we need to yield.

I have reached the point that I can live in another country, away from my spouse, knowing that we are both living our lives according to our own purposes and that we will come together when we are supposed to.

When we let go of trying to control people and situations, we feel very free because, in the long run, we can only control ourselves. It is the same when we have an opinion about something. If we try to convince others, we expend a lot of energy. They may have an opinion that is completely different from ours, but, if we are secure in ourselves, it doesn't matter. We do not have to control the situation. Our main objective should be to find a way to live, without shame and guilt, honoring our own path. To be true to ourselves, to honor our

Spirit and purpose on earth, we need to do only what is right for us. How then, do we develop happy relationships?

The Key to Happy Relationships

What is the key to happy relationships? Working as a counselor for many years, I see relationships as they are crumbling and I have noticed the same patterns over and over again. What appears to be happening is that they have reached an impasse, a breakdown in communication that they can't get past.

The breakdown is usually over something very small which escalated to something big. Normally it is some expectation that is not being met. The one party wants something from the other person, which they don't get. It could be more attention or more involvement from the other person. For example, I have seen couples in open hostility because neither one feels loved. It is obvious to me, as an onlooker, that the love exists but both partners remain locked in recrimination and blame. Since we choose partners who are similar to parental figures, we often recreate these situations by choosing someone who imitates the rejecting behavior of our parents.

I remind clients, however, that the relationship is a gift because it allows you to look at the unhealed parts of yourself. When you react to the other party with so much emotion, you know that this emotion is attached to early memories that remain unhealed within yourself.

How do we heal ourselves so that we don't repeat old dysfunctional patterns in one relationship after another and end up saying that we don't want a relationship at all? The first thing that is important is a healthy expression of emotions. We have to open the process of communication so that we can express our needs and how we feel. If it is too difficult to do this, often it is helpful to have a therapist or third party available to clarify the communication at first. We will always have disagreement in our relationships, but we have to find a constructive way of expressing it.

We need to eliminate the need for conflict. A relationship is like a game of tennis and when one person fails to hit the ball back, the game is over. It is very hard for one person to fight alone. How do you learn to stop hitting the ball back? The two most important qualities in a relationship, I have found, are non-judgment and forgiveness. I like to look at non-judgment in an Eastern way. Influenced by both Taoism and Buddhism, this kind of non-judgment rests on the understanding that everyone is here following their own path, working out their karma. We cannot judge anyone's situation because we don't understand the whole picture.

How do you not judge when people have said very nasty things to you or treated you badly and you are still holding a grievance against them? Not judging is like seeing yourself in a play together and each of you is playing your part. Try to concentrate on just what is coming up for you. What can I learn from this? Is this a pattern? When do I feel these things? It is very hard to do from the worldly framework because we get caught up in the drama of it. This is when practices, such as the ones that I will give you later on, help us quiet our minds for a while so we can connect with the more spiritual side of ourselves.

Forgiveness also needs the same kind of removal from the world. Forgiveness, as we have known it, is the forgetting of things that really bother us. It is trying to put out of our minds things that we perceive have been done to us. The problem with this kind of forgiveness is that we don't really manage to keep things out of our mind. Some action will bring up something from the past and we still feel the same feelings. We bury the feelings but they are still there.

Spiritual forgiveness is seeing beyond the worldly significance of the situation, knowing that there is something we are to learn. It is knowing that everyone is just playing his or her part and there is nothing to forgive. The interaction is just giving us more awareness of our own patterns.

We need to express our emotions in a way that does not damage our relationships. The drama that exists in most relationships creates an atmosphere of turbulence most of the time.

The first thing you have to eliminate is the need for drama. Why would we need drama in our life? Consciously we probably would not want it, but unconsciously it feels familiar so we attract it. We have to change our consciousness so that peace

31

starts to feel more familiar. We will look at this need more in the next section.

In my case, it meant moving away and living by myself for a while. In the beginning, I would crave some kind of excited communication but, after a while, I only wanted peace. When my husband would come to visit and we would get into the old argument pattern, I would know that it no longer belonged in my life and, when I did not participate, things would improve as a result.

The spiritual literature points out that we cannot link with Spirit if we are immersed in drama. We need a quiet mind to be clear enough to receive our spiritual guidance. As we start to be more in touch with Spirit, we realize that all those conflicts were lessons for us and most of the things we were fighting existed in ourselves. As we become aware of and release the old patterns, we find a new peaceful way of living which gives us more satisfaction. The things that used to bother us do not. When our partner or someone else starts an interaction which would normally bring an angry reaction in us, we look at them and realize that their behavior has nothing to do with us. We might have triggered it but it has to do with their reaction to an early relationship in their life. They are arguing with their mother, father or a sibling. We all recreate these situations in our life.

We feel so free when we realize this fact, and, even though the feelings are intense, we start to notice old patterns and we back off. It is very necessary to have practices which calm the mind. When we attain a quiet mind, we look within and and notice the chaos, realize the old pattern and maybe even feel the intensity of that time and let it go.

Once you get used to a feeling of peace, you cannot go back to the old chaos. It will remain foreign to you. Once you have released the chaos, you will start to attract peaceful situations into your life. The old arguments and conflicts will be a thing of the past. You will truly be living the qualities of this part of the bagua—yielding, receptivity, openness and trust.

Relationship Exercise

Think about a person who is causing you difficulties now. I suggest getting quiet and, in your mind, take yourself back to a time when you felt this highly emotional state before. I am sure you will remember a time in your childhood. See the person in front of you with whom you feel similar debilitating emotions. It may be your mother or father or some one else in your early life. You may spend some time exploring these feelings. Do not be afraid to connect with them.

As you stand there as that child, see that other person transform into a child. You are both children standing together. What kind of child was this person? Probably you will see that this child was not a happy one and was having many difficulties. Feel yourself the more resilient child and, in your imagination, encourage this other child to play with you. That might be very difficult to do. Imagine yourself playing with this child, showing him or her some happy childhood games.

As you feel yourself both children, you get in touch with the early conditioning of the person who caused you the problems. You find that it is difficult to get mad at this child because he or she is acting in a conditioned way. Imagine yourself hugging that child and saying that you understand the behavior and you know now that it has nothing to do with you. Picture a light surrounding that child, acknowledging the higher presence that he or she may not be aware of. Thank this person for playing this difficult role in your life, helping you to be aware of your own patterns. This type of forgiveness affirms that we all have a divine role of which we may not be aware. Whenever you are in conflict with someone, take some time to do this exercise. You will find that it changes your view of this person.

Affirmations

I have loving, supportive relationships in my life.

I have a loving partnership with a significant other in my life.

I nurture others and allow myself to be nurtured.

I acknowledge the higher presence of all the people in my life.

Feng Shui for Your Environment

This part of the bagua is the place to build relationships and partnerships. Suggestions for this area include:

- Things that symbolize a relationship to you
- A picture of lovers
- Round shapes (representing earth) or square (representing relationships) shapes
- A pair of anything - hearts, doves, birds etc.
- A pair of chairs with receptive pillows
- The colors of pink as well as earth tones
- A hanging plant flowing down

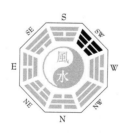

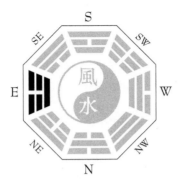

Chapter 3

Ancestors

Ancestors Trigram

This trigram, called "chen," is symbolized by a strong yang line pushing upward below two unbroken yin lines. The trigram means "shocking thunder" and has often been represented by a dragon soaring out of the depths into stormy skies. In the archetypal family, it is the eldest son. The element is wood, which refers to rising energy as in spring when trees burst into life. The color is spring green.

In Feng Shui, this is the trigram associated with ancestors or what came before. It is on the East side of your house. Just as things burst into blossom in spring, we must move forward in our lives. How we move forward depends on where we have been before. How we interpret the messages that have been passed on to us over time from our ancestral roots creates our future. In the bagua, this trigram is across from the trigram of creativity, projects or offspring. How we deal with what came before determines our progeny, whether people or things.

In this chapter we will look at releasing clutter or old energy from our lives and at some of the out-dated family messages still influencing our lives, as well as what we can learn from our ancestors and the elders of our society.

Letting Go

Before we can do Feng Shui on our environment, we must let go of all clutter. Wherever we accumulate clutter, we have dead or stagnant energy, as well as blocks in the free flow of energy.

When we do Feng Shui, we have to take a close look at our environment and decide what things need to be released in order to let the energy circulate freely. Whatever we do in our milieu will also translate into our lives, and vice versa. As we let go of clutter in our surroundings, we will also start to feel free emotionally. As we start to heal old emotional wounds, we will want to have clarity in our environments.

Why do we hold onto clutter? Whatever we have in our environments is synonymous with the clutter we hold in our lives generally. We accumulate clutter in case we might need something again. It is that fear of giving up the past.

Often we have a sentimental attachment to things of the past and we want to keep mementos of them to remind ourselves of these things. By doing this, we keep ourselves in old energy patterns which impede us from moving forward.

Sometimes we have purchased something that is very expensive and we feel guilt about letting it go. We are tied to our rationalizations that we will find a use for it sometime. For years I held onto very expensive handbags, shoes and clothing that I had purchased on trips and had not worn. Wherever I moved, I brought them with me, hoping that I would find some use for them. After studying Feng Shui, I gave them away to people who appreciated them. Now I give things away as soon as I find no use for them and feel the accompanying freeing up of energy that occurs.

We identify with possessions in our lives and sometimes they make a statement of who we are. It is hard for us to let go of valued belongings because it feels like we are giving up part of ourselves. Sometimes these possessions, like an expensive outfit, provide status for us. Often they are associated with someone else; for instance, something we have inherited that we cannot give up because we feel that giving it up is letting go of our tie to the benefactor.

In a strange way possessions can create security for us and, as long as we are surrounded by "stuff," we feel secure. Some of us feel nervous about empty spaces and we feel cushioned against anything that might happen to us. In the same way, many of us hold on to eating patterns that keep us overweight. We feel cushioned and protected against the pain of having to deal with old issues, especially in relationships. We hold on to deep emotional hurts because we are afraid of the pain of looking at them again. Ironically, the surfacing or revisiting of these emotions gives us the opportunity to release the old hurts and move past them.

It is the same with clutter in our environment. We keep ourselves surrounded by things as a way of suppressing our emotions and keeping ourselves overwhelmed. It is that unconscious need for struggle that keeps us from being fully alive.

These are all patterns that have developed from our childhood in the same way as the patterns in relationships discussed in the last chapter. These messages, like in the trigram, soar from the depths of our buried memories, holding us back from moving forward in our lives.

As we clear our environment, we will encounter the residue of patterns in our lives that are holding us back. To be truly free in our lives, we must face these patterns and move through them.

Out-dated Messages Holding Us Back

As I clear out the clutter from my house, I am aware of things that I have accumulated which signify old patterns in my life. The most common patterns that I see in myself and others are holding onto struggle, shame, guilt, and chaos.

Life is a Struggle

As I go through my possessions, I get in touch with the feeling of being overwhelmed. I have been going in so many directions in my career and, as a result, I have the residue all over my house. The many courses I have taught over the years as well as my many business investments and their accompanying legal documents clutter my drawers and filing cabinets.

I have cabinets for Canadian business as well as for American business. Since I sell products, I have boxes of items in different places in my house. As I clear out my clutter, I realize that my need for so many things in my life is related to my old pattern of believing "life is a struggle."

We show this by feeling weighed down as though everything is a burden. I see this pattern manifested in my clients as not being able to feel any joy in anything, of feeling the weight of the world on their shoulders.

Most people develop this feeling when they are children. When I was a child, I felt this message from my father who had lived through the Depression and World War II and, even though he was a dentist, had had a lot of financial difficulties. He talked about the times that he had to do dentistry for a bag of potatoes during the 1930s. Even though things improved for him, he kept that feeling buried but it was manifested many times in many ways.

He made it clear through his actions, if not verbally, that it was not all right to enjoy things. When I would be having fun playing as a child, he would stop it somewhere along the line, making it clear that life was serious and not to be enjoyed. He had a good sense of humor but there was another side of him which surfaced soon after his laughter, to make sure that he did not have fun too long.

Reading old diaries of his father who had been a schoolteacher and writer of history books and then, after returning to college, a dentist, I see the old message of seriousness reoccurring. He was very influenced by the Temperance Movement at the time and having fun and frivolity were associated with drinking which, for him, was the work of the devil.

He writes a very sad account of my grandmother having a stroke and becoming nasty and abusive and eventually having to be put in a home where she died. My grandfather tried to look after her but could not and, in the process, got sick himself. When my father was a teenager, he looked after his father until he died and even somehow felt responsible for his death.

Set on his own at an early age with all those painful memories of both his parents' deaths was not an easy thing for my father to get over and, not having the awareness that we do these days, he never did. In these old diaries, I sense an overwhelming sadness and heaviness in the home where my father was brought up and he had these buried feelings all his life. He would show a lot of emotion, usually anger, but also a deep buried sadness.

My sister's death at the age of 25 was a tremendous blow to my father. She was a bright star who had made exceptional accomplishments at her age. She was extremely intelligent and had walked through a master's degree at a young age with top honors. She was also an accomplished musician and my father, a musician himself, was very proud of her. His life wrapped around her and, even after she had left home, he would wait eagerly for her short return visits with many of her interesting and famous friends. While in the diplomatic service in Malaysia, her life ended in a tragic accident. She fell to her death over a waterfall while mountain climbing in an unknown terrain. Both my parents were devastated but my father never got over his sadness and bitterness. His heaviness increased in his later years.

My mother, on the other hand, was very business-like and showed very little emotion. Her anger would come out on occasion and I had been told that she was a very stern teacher in her day but, as a parent, she was reasonable and fairly balanced. I got the feeling from her side of the family that her home had been devoid of emotion. Her father's job changed many times and she moved on many occasions. I felt that her modus operandi was not to get too close in case you didn't see the person again. You could feel the emotion behind her competent exterior and it would leak out on many occasions. It, too, was a sadness which was accentuated after my sister's death.

The result of living in this household was that joy was infrequent and, when I was too happy, I felt guilty. I was 21 when my sister died and, even if it was not stated by my parents, I was left with the feeling that I had to make up for her death. One of my parent's friends even told me that I had to carry on for my sister (Mary) now. This, along with the feeling of burden that I already had from my home, added tremendous weight to my life.

Because of this conditioning, I often feel the weight of having to do something even before I do it. I have found that, if I have a lot of tasks to do, they feel overwhelming and I can hardly get myself motivated to do them. I also know that I create these tasks on a subconscious level.

Even as a child, I remember the feeling of having to do many tasks around the house before we, the family, could enjoy ourselves. When I got my first home with my husband and children, my parents would visit and show me all the things which needed to be done. Because I had been brought up that way, I believed that these tasks needed to be done by me. Consequently, it was hard for me to enjoy my house because I was always aware of the enormous amount of work waiting for me. I was also going back to school and had endless studies to do on top of supervising the lives of two young kids.

Later, I invested in a number of properties which all required work and burdensome mortgage payments as well as a business which had heavy bills and employees to pay. It never occurred to me, at that time, that I had a choice to live in a manner which was light and free. Even now, I am still freeing my life by unloading properties and mortgages and innumerable burdens that I had taken on.

As I became more aware of Feng Shui and the need to release clutter, I realized that I did have a choice—that it was acceptable to live free without many possessions and obligations to worry about. Many of us are so used to the burdens and the accompanying worry that it feels normal to us. I see people who walk into my office, complaining that their lives are not fulfilled. As they sit in the chair, I see that holding burdens is one of their problems because they look as if they are carrying a bag of bricks on their back.

These people have usually taken on other peoples' problems,

often their families,' and they hold on to their problems as if they were their own. We cannot carry other peoples' burdens but we try to carry them anyway. If only their lives would improve, then ours would lighten, we think. However, since this is our unconscious mind at work, we would create other burdens if we didn't have theirs. I see clients who have given up complete control of their happiness and put it into the hands of relatives, spouses or friends. "When they get their act together, I will be free," they will say.

I try to point out that this feeling was established in childhood. We learned as children to take care of family members. Unconsciously we have developed a feeling of responsibility for others. This happens often when parents are alcoholics or appear not to be able to take care of themselves. Another pattern, which emerges frequently, is feeling shame.

SHAME

Have you ever felt that you don't belong where you are and maybe you've had that feeling most of your life? Maybe when you were a child, you didn't quite fit into a certain group of playmates. Maybe you felt somehow lonely even in a crowd. You might have experienced in very early childhood humiliating experiences that made you feel like a misfit.

When I look back at my childhood, I spent a lot of time looking from the sidelines, not quite fitting in. In kindergarten, I was painfully shy and used to be afraid to approach other kids. I was not like a lot of other children I saw who were aggressive and could walk into a crowd of kids and fit right in. I would observe and then be afraid to approach. Inadvertently, through their disapproval, my parents had instilled in me a sense of being ashamed of myself, and strict teachers reinforced that feeling. My lack of confidence gave me a feeling that I would not be accepted. I had some playmates near my home, but it took me a long time to find children to play with at school.

When I did find children to talk to at school, I would talk to them in class and get punished for it. I remember a particularly painful incident in which I was sent into the corner facing the wall at the back of the classroom as punishment for talking. Incidents like that can leave indelible marks on your subconscious and the feelings can stay with you all your life.

This feeling manifests as shame and most of us have it. Frequently it comes upon us from almost nowhere. We are in a situation that triggers that old feeling of humiliation and, all of a sudden, we have that wash of old emotion come to us. Sometimes we wake up in the morning with that feeling in the pit of our stomach.

The esoteric literature tells us that this was one of the feelings engrained in us from lifetime to lifetime. Those of us who are spiritually aware and believe in other lifetimes, believe that we were probably shamed and maybe even killed for our belief systems in other incarnations. As we look back in history, we know that many people were punished for their beliefs in many countries in the world, including the United States, up to very recent years.

This shame is buried at the cellular level of your body and, as it comes up to be released, you may be feeling it even stronger. Those feelings, if repressed, are the ones which make people strike out at other people. The more we condemn or try to punish other people, the more we are feeling badly about ourselves. What we dislike in another is usually a part of ourselves that we don't want to look at. To be really self-aware, we need to recognize the feelings that we have inside us. The Ancestors trigram reminds us to release these old messages in order to be free.

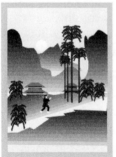

Another message that is engrained in a lot of us from an early age is guilt.

Guilt

Our society has a lot of rules and, if we don't follow them, we are shamed and made to feel guilty. We feel guilty if we do quite natural things; we feel like we are doing something wrong when we do things we enjoy.

In the same way we learn these other patterns, we learn that some things are acceptable and others are not, and our social culture, whether it is our family or friends, lets us know when we have strayed from the norm.

Mothers are blamed for making children feel guilty, often for something as simple as toilet training. Children are taught very early that they should feel guilty for many things, the same things that we, as mothers, felt guilty about. I believe that is often why children rebel.

I see many children who are labeled emotionally disturbed and I can sense a great deal of frustration in them. We are asking these children to stop doing things that feel perfectly natural, like talking to one another and moving around, and they show this frustration through anger. Instead of working with their innate instincts, we expect them to stay in one place and be perfectly silent.

When I go into a school and see children having violent temper tantrums, I know that they may have been thwarted in every attempt at doing what feels natural to them. They often rebel against what appears to them to be unreasonable discipline.

This pattern of feeling guilty can continue all our life. In my case, my father told me that I was not to talk back to him or express any anger. Also, as I said before, I was not to feel much joy, either. The result was that I spent a lot of my younger years feeling guilty for feeling anything.

This manifested itself, in later years, as a vague sense of guilt around anything I did. I would do it anyway, but I could not enjoy anything fully. I still fight with guilt when I am taking time off from my work or having too much fun.

Even excessive weight can be related to a feeling of guilt. At mealtime, I'm sure that you were told that there were many starving people and you should not throw away food. There are many overweight people I see now in therapy who unconsciously feel guilty if they don't eat everything on their plate. These feelings and other buried patterns often keep us attracting chaos into our lives.

The Need for Chaos

Many of us have been brought up in an environment where there was a lot of conflict, fighting and general confusion. We have become accustomed to this type of environment and it feels familiar. Unconsciously we are attracted to it whether we know it or not. If we have a lot of confusion in our working life or our home life, it is because we have unconsciously drawn it to us. On the surface we may not like it, but we can function in it nevertheless.

I was brought up in a home with a father who could never be satisfied with anything. The way that he demonstrated this was a short temper that he displayed at least once, if not several times, each day. As a dentist, he would not show it with his patients but he would take out the frustration that he felt over late or missed appointments or money problems on his family.

I learned that I could set off that temper with many little things that I did and said and, sometimes to feel rebellious, I would set off that temper consciously. Generally though, the atmosphere when he was around was like a minefield. You never knew when you would set off an explosion. The result was that I would walk around him as if I were treading on eggs, being afraid to step too hard in case one broke.

My mother was subtler about the things that upset her. She also was very touchy but she would show her disapproval in a more nonverbal way. I knew, by looking at the expression on her face, that I had done something wrong. As a child, you somehow feel that you are responsible for your parents' anger, that you caused it and it is up to you to make it better.

In addition to guilt, I got used to being judged as bad and having chaotic feelings going on inside me all the time. As I got into relationships later on, I would bring people into my life which would duplicate those feelings of chaos. Unconsciously, I would create an environment of conflict and argument.

The end result is constant turmoil, interspersed with calm and loving times, which seem to make up for the conflict. However, blame and argument come up very fast whenever there is anything out of place. Children who grow up in that type of home learn to react in the same way and create it in their later years. We call this syndrome the need for drama which is part of many families. But how do we clear out these patterns?

Clearing Away Old Patterns

Clearing out my houses as I have moved out of them, I have seen the residue of patterns in my life that have to be released. As I simplify my life and my possessions, I feel a certain freedom that I want to maintain. I recognize that, many times before, I have cleared out clutter but, very soon, have burdened my life again with possessions and obligations. To move forward in our lives, we have to deal with the consciousness that creates this burden.

Remember that the power of Feng Shui is to analyze our lives by looking at the symbols around us. We have created these symbols because they define who we are. When we look at the symbols around us, we ask ourselves whether they truly represent who we want to be. If not, let us look at changing them.

When we are surrounded by things that we do not like and which do not feel good any more, our energy drops. If we surround ourselves by the things we love, we start to feel peace in our lives.

We all have the right to live free from burdens and clutter. In fact, we cannot be helpful to others while we are carrying burdens. When we think of clutter, it includes our environments, possessions, work and relationships. Have we accumulated clutter in these areas? Are we in outmoded relationships that do not empower us? Are we in work that no longer serves us?

For me, analyzing the symbols helped me to understand what was going on in my life. As I began to clear my environment, I saw too many possessions around my house, too many clothes in my closet, and too much of all kinds of work waiting to be done. Also, I was aware of too many obligations and commitments to people. I saw that these things all contributed to a feeling of being overwhelmed.

I started with my closet and began to eliminate clothing which did not suit my present image. I had many things which did not feel right any more. As we undergo transformation, we start to exude a new energy that requires us to look different from before.

I began to give away possessions that represented other times in my life. I kept only those things that represented me in my present state.

As I surveyed my many obligations, I realized that there were some things I was doing that I did not enjoy any more. I asked the question "Does this bring me joy any more?" If not, I found a graceful way of removing it from my life. I resigned from many clubs and committees.

Was I doing work for money or the joy of doing it? I started to ask myself if I really wanted to spend time doing these things. I started to concentrate mainly on things that make me feel good, although they were not bringing as much money. I knew that money would come over time.

I stepped back from my relationships and asked whether some of them were draining my energy. I have pulled away from relationships that were troublesome. I looked at the lesson that I had to learn and lovingly moved on, leaving those people free to learn their own lessons.

All the esoteric literature points out that we cannot link with Spirit if we are immersed in drama, that we have to give up those patterns in order to be clear enough to receive spiritual guidance.

As we realize that conflicts are lessons for us and most of the things we are fighting are inside ourselves, we find a new peaceful way of living. Once you have that feeling of tranquility and order, you cannot go back to the old chaos. It will remain foreign to you and you will start to attract more peaceful situations.

As we clear out the past, it is important to be aware of where we have been. As we move on, we are becoming older and wiser and having more to contribute to society, as we share our experiences with others. This is the trigram which reminds us that there is a lot to learn from our ancestors and the elders of our society.

Respect for the Elderly

Through my connections, when I visited Hong Kong I spent a lot of time going out socially with Chinese families. The feeling that I got was familiar, one that I remember when I was around Chinese students years ago. It was a feeling of deep respect and honor. There is a depth of feeling which is hard to find in North American culture. Since these people were told by their American relatives to treat me like family, there was a sense that they went out of their way to accommodate me. When I did things for them, there was a deep appreciation. The Chinese also respect education and honor the process of aging.

What is the feeling of connectedness which exists among these people? In Hong Kong, in particular, where families often co-exist in small surroundings, they must find a way to get along. They are also taught from childhood, to honor their elders and the wisdom acquired with age.

That is something very lacking in our society. Our culture is youth-oriented and we think that older people are out-dated and have nothing to offer us. My father used to say, "Our generation is on the firing line." He meant by this that his generation was dying off and was not honored any more than a line of people waiting for execution.

As I get older, I understand this sentiment somewhat. Now that I have lived longer and have a deeper perspective from all my experiences, I find that my age and experience are not necessarily honored by the youth.

What I pick up in Chinese culture is a respect for the aging process. From their ancient culture, which has eroded somewhat today, comes the understanding that longevity goes hand in hand with wisdom. In our culture, I fight feelings of getting older, of getting past my prime, longing for the youthful body of years before. Especially for women, societal pressure tells us to try hard to keep our face and body youthful in appearance. Some of us even go to the extreme of having body tucks and face-lifts.

On the other hand, as I use my Qigong practices and understand my proper place in this universe, I know that, in terms of intellect and wisdom, I am reaching my prime. Even physically, these practices are increasing my vitality and longevity.

In the indigenous tribes, it is the elders who raise the children, teaching them from the perspective of wisdom gained from living all those years. Our society has to honor the aging process. From an earthly perspective, we get older and wiser. From a spiritual perspective, we never age. In fact, there is no such thing as aging. We have something timeless and ageless in ourselves that we can access.

We are so taken up in our everyday experiences that we forget why we are really here. One way of getting in touch with this part of ourselves is respecting that element in other people. When we concentrate on the goodness in others, we get a sense of the community of man.

We look past the crassness, the loudness, and even the violence of others and say silently to them, "You do not know who you are but I know you are a spiritual being." There is a sense of respect and honor when you do this and it returns to you. I feel it from my Chinese friends. Their actions are beyond knowledge. It is as if there is an ancient encoding that speaks inside them of which even they are not aware. They remind us, through parts of their culture, that there are valuable messages of peace, harmony, sacredness and reverence gained from the past.

Messages from the Ancestors

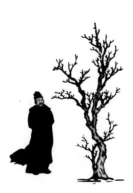

There are messages from even the elderly who no longer appear to be functional in our society. As I sit in a nursing home with my mother who is now 94 years of age, in a wheel chair, and unaware of her surroundings, I think about what the meaning of life is for her and other residents.

It does not seem that people in that condition have much to contribute now, but I know that they have an unstated message for the rest of us. My mother has become very angelic in these years and, although unaware of who people are, is very pleasant and complimentary to the workers in the home. She has flash-backs to the past but the memories of her early years are selective and pleasant.

There are others in the home who seem to be tormented by the past and spend their days swearing, hitting out and hurling abusive messages to the staff and visitors. As a psychologist, I think about what early experiences remain in their subconscious minds to bring about such violent reactions. I believe that these people are still very influenced by problems unresolved in their lifetime. My mother and some others like her seem to have gone past the personality issues and are influenced more by Spirit at this time.

We keep the elderly alive much longer because of modern medicine, but there must be a spiritual reason why they are still here. What are the messages they have for us?

For one, the message I receive is for us to work through these emotional issues in our early years, so they will not torment us later on. What has been buried surfaces at crucial times and remains with you until you clear it. These early influences were ignored by the elderly of this generation and they lived their lives never looking at the depth of these feelings. I have seen these older women and men reenacting early conflicts with brothers, sisters and parents. They also suppressed their regrets and remorse for not taking risks in their earlier years and these feel-ings boil up from their subconscious now. Even though many of them are close to their death, they have not come to terms with their lives and have no sense of peace.

The message from those who, like my mother, have gone beyond those early experiences, is to live entirely in the present. My mother is not aware of the past or future. She is dealing only with what is happening to her at this time. The torments of the past are over and she has no concern for the future. If we could only live our lives this way, we would be connected with the guid-ance of Spirit as it exists within us. I often have the feeling, when

I am with my mother, that she is hearing the voice of Spirit more and thus remaining content and happy.

What would I have missed if I had not had this experience with my mother, if she had not survived into this period of her life? What has been the message for me? In her early years, she had always been interested in money and possessions. When she first got sick, I showed her the diamond ring, which had meant a lot to her, and she looked at it without even a sign of recognition. For years she had refused to give up her house because her father had built it. After she got sick, she did not even remember her house. The message here is to completely detach from our possessions because they mean nothing in the long run. We cannot take them with us.

The messages of these older people confined in nursing homes are more for the staff and visitors. They are living for us, not themselves. I have never seen such patience and compassion as exhibited by the caregivers in this nursing home and in others where I have been. The residents have become children again and they need total care. The staff who take care of them do so in a way that is beyond the money they receive for this job. The elderly make us take a look at our lives and think about how we can gracefully move into old age.

They make us look at how we can bring peace into our lives and disconnect from worldly pursuits. They make us remember our ancestral roots, as well as what we can contribute to the next generation.

Clearing the Past Exercise

Take a deep breath and get in a quiet state while you ask yourself these questions.

Do you feel burdened by situations and people? If so, how do you feel this burden? Often we feel it as heaviness in our mood and actions. In our body, we often have tension through our shoulders or back, as if we were holding the weight of the world on our back.

Do you feel shame easily? Start to be aware of the times you feel this emotion. It no doubt goes back to an early time in your life.

Do you often feel guilt? As in the last one, be aware of when you feel this and relate it to an early period of your life.

Take a look at your environment. What is it telling you about what is going on in your life? Do you have to release possessions, obligations, burdens, and even some relationships?

Do you still attract chaos in your life? Are you willing to see that there is a more peaceful way to live?

Visualize a situation that normally brings guilt, shame, chaos or struggle. Create a scene in your mind that brings one or all of these responses, noticing the trigger that creates the usual reaction. We are going to learn to choose another response.

Get a picture in your mind of yourself in a former situation in which you were completely relaxed and calm. If you cannot relate to a situation, imagine a time like this. Make this scene as real as possible. Picture what you are wearing, what you are seeing, what you are hearing, even touching, tasting and smelling. The more you involve your senses and the more real you make this scene, the easier it is to create in your life.

Whenever you feel the old conditioned response, bring into your mind immediately this peaceful scene. The more you do this, the more you are allowing the old feelings to be replaced by the new calm reaction. Allow yourself to feel the pride and satisfaction that you receive as you move past the old conditioned response. If you do this regularly, you are creating a new and powerful response.

Affirmations

I release burden from my life.

I release shame and guilt.

I release chaos from my life.

I use the helpful messages from the past to guide me in the present.

Feng Shui for Your Environment

This is the part of your home to emphasize ancestors or helpful messages from the past. The element is wood. Suggestions here are:

- Pictures of parents or ancestors
- Symbols or pictures of any person from the past whose life has meaning to you now
- Anything made of wood and columnar or tubular shapes, such as pillars
- Floral prints, striped cloth which all represent wood
- The color of green
- Plants or pictures of trees or forests

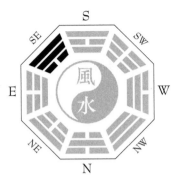

CHAPTER 4
WEALTH

Wealth Trigram

The trigram for wealth, "Sun," is 2 unbroken lines above a single broken line. In terms of the archetypal family, it represents the oldest daughter. This trigram symbolizes persistent wind and consistent penetration. It represents the gradual accumulation of wealth with patience and self-control. It is the element of wood, and the colors are the color of wood—brown and green—as well as purple, which blends the green of the ancestors trigram and the red of the fame trigram. It is the Southeast corner of your house.

On the bagua, it is opposite helpful people and the two concepts are very related. The accumulation of wealth usually has to do with help from others and helping others by giving money or supporting their growth in other ways. The concept of wealth refers not only to money but to blessings of all kinds.

In this area, I will look at what abundance means, how we deal with wealth and prosperity, the fears and patterns which hold us back from achieving it, and how we can give up the path of struggle and become magnetic to abundance.

Abundance is a State of Mind

Many of us think that our problems would disappear if we had more money. No matter how important money may be, it is just one form of abundance. Abundance is a state of mind. It includes inner peace and a feeling of having plenty of time, love and every other good thing—including money.

In order to achieve this state of mind, we have to release the rigid conditioning which holds us in lack and limitation. Since money is the most obvious form of abundance, let us take a closer look at money to see what it reveals to us about our mind-set.

Money plays a very important part in our life because there is very little that we can do without it. It is necessary for our existence but, as a result, we have a lot of strong feelings about money. In fact, a study done years ago by a research department of a major university found that money was what people worried about the most; it was also what made people the happiest - and the unhappiest.

What is money really? It is the means of exchange that the world has devised to render goods and services. Money has no value in itself, however. What gives it importance is the value we assign to it. We chase after it in order to fulfill our desires which usually means amassing "things."

Because it is so ingrained in all cultures, we spend a great deal of time dealing with money, either getting it or spending it. Almost every day we have some transaction, buying something at the store, selling something or earning money through our work. Therefore, we have a strong emotional tie to money and have strong feelings toward it, even if they are subconscious. It is necessary to surface all these feelings because they tell us a lot about ourselves.

How do we develop our feelings about money? In this world, it is easy to feel that we are at the mercy of the economic system.

We think that we do not have power over making our own money, that it can be ripped away from us at any time because of economic crashes, recessions etc. In fact, the general thinking of the populace creates recessions. The stock market, for example, goes up and down with the perceptions of people about decisions of political leaders, business and world conditions.

Also, we are bombarded by the negative thinking of people around us. We hear clichés and comments such as, "If you aren't careful, you will lose all your money" or " Money is limited." or "Money doesn't grow on trees" or "Save your pennies for a rainy day." The philosophy of our society dictates lack of all kinds.

I believe that we deal with money the way we deal with life. If we are stingy with money, we are stingy in the way we live our life. Those who are afraid to spend their money also tend to live a very limited existence without enjoying themselves or giving fully of themselves in relationships.

If we are afraid that we will lose our money, even if we are wealthy, we hold onto other things in our life the same way, especially our emotions. I knew a woman who was very wealthy but was always afraid that she would lose her money. She eventually died in her forties of colon cancer, a disease related to the pattern of repressing emotions.

A lot of us let our feelings of self worth go up and down with our ability to make money. If we have a good job and we make a lot of money, we feel that we must be worthy because society values us for what we do. Even then, we deal with feelings of unworthiness buried deep in our subconscious which we know have nothing to do with accumulating money.

Men, especially, are told that their worth depends on the type of job they have and the money they earn. Since both men and women with good jobs and material wealth are not necessarily happy, we, as a society, are starting to question the value of this thinking. What we can learn from our ability to attract and keep money are old emotional patterns that exist within us.

If you are aware of your feelings about money today, you will see reflected the ideas that you heard expressed by your parents or the other people around you, as well as the way they acted around money. These early impressions get stored in the subconscious mind and any time we run into a familiar situation the old patterns of reacting automatically occur. For example, if we were brought up with parents who worried about money at Christmas, we might start to feel that concern triggered each Christmas, even though we now have money.

How did your parents feel about and talk about money? Was it something they perceived as coming to them freely or was it something they believed they struggled to get? Did they talk freely about money or was it a forbidden topic? Was it associated with aliveness, happiness, well being and self-love, or was it associated with burdens and problems?

Those of us who are still struggling with money issues usually have been conditioned with the mind-set that money is a burden, that it is difficult to get and that we do not deserve to have it. In addition to what we heard from our parents, this idea is reflected in most of society to day. There are also common fears associated with money.

Fears and Patterns Associated with Money

The most common fears are fear of failure, fear of success, fear of rejection, fear of death, fear of the unknown and fear of loss.

Fear of failure can keep you from going into your own business or doing anything that puts yourself on the line. Conversely, you may do rash things which do not work, not admitting to having this fear.

Fear of success is usually denied and suppressed, but one indicator of it is jealousy or envy of people who are successful. You may find that you are full of excuses about why you can't succeed or you sabotage yourself when you do get some success or get close to having success.

Fear of rejection often comes about if we have to sell a product or our own services. Because of this fear, we often stay in situations in which we never have to extend ourselves. We might stay in jobs that we dislike and never try anything which might be more challenging.

Making money is referred to as "making a living," so being without it can be equated to death. This innate fear allows us to do anything to get money, including staying in a job that we hate.

If you have fear of the unknown, you may never take a risk or make any changes in your life so you can remain safe. Fear of loss can also keep you from launching any new venture, especially in business, but also in life generally.

Shame about money is also a pattern—shame about not having enough, having more than other people, or desiring to have money at all. Sometimes we have learned, from our parents or our religious institutions, that it is wrong to have a lot of money. The famous adage "money is the root of all evil" is misquoted because it was "the love of money is the root of all evil." It is our attitude toward money that is important.

We show our general patterns in life around money issues more than anything else. If we feel powerless in our life, we will create situations that put other people in control of our money. Also, we might make risky investments that we have no control over and often end up losing our money.

In the same vain, we create an "I am a victim" mentality and get involved in businesses that leave us in the control of others. When things go bad in the business, we find ourselves at the mercy of other people's decisions and feel victimized by those people.

The "life is a struggle" mentality keeps us always fighting to make money and to keep it. We choose ways of making money that keep us in the "struggle mode." One of the places that this struggle mentality is most evident is in the accumulation of debt.

If you are struggling with a lack of money in your life today, it is probably because of one or more of these patterns. Let us take a closer look at debt as an example of how these patterns can be perpetuated.

Debt

There is no more obvious a place for the pattern of "life is a struggle" than the concept of debt. With the introduction of credit cards and, even before that, mortgages, many of us in this culture are in debt. We have grown used to being able to pay for things quickly and easily and worry about how we will get the money later on.

Unfortunately what happens often is that we don't get the money later on and we keep paying the credit cards' minimum monthly balance or the interest on the mortgage and never pay them off. Our life becomes a vicious cycle with the money that we are earning going out to pay monthly interest payments.

What happens to many is that they get so burdened by these monthly payments that they eventually have to declare bankruptcy in order to get some relief. This is becoming more and more frequent.

I believe that debt is more than a belief in having everything fast (immediate gratification). More often, it is an underlying philosophy that exists inside most of us. We have learned that life is a struggle and that being submerged by obligations feels like the way that we should live.

For generations, hard work and toil have been exemplified as the way to live and, if we are not living that way, we should feel vaguely guilty. For most of us, even though we pay off one debt, we will soon amass another one.

I know a lot about this because I have been caught in this credit card struggle for many years. It seemed like the natural way to pay for things when I went into business, but I did not realize that I was putting myself in a hole. I have paid off my debt many times but always took on more, usually for business related things that I felt were necessary.

I have always felt so free when I paid everything off, but soon would take on more debts and feel weighed under again. Subconsciously I became so used to the notion of struggle that it felt unnatural without it. It is similar to what happens in a relationship when we are used to conflict in our earlier years. We say that we don't like conflict but, until we become aware of our pattern, we will create it over and over again.

How do we get out of this endless cycle of debt? I do not believe that destroying all credit cards will do anything to change our pattern. As we learn to change out mind-set, we will be able to use them responsibly.

Our whole culture is based on consumption of energy, whether it be our fast-paced society, our excessive emotional responses or the emphasis on consumerism. We are taught to consume energy, not to conserve it. The Taoist practices introduced in this book will help us conserve and build our energy so we have plenty to expend when we need it.

In the same way, we can conserve and build the energy of money, but we first have to believe that it, too, is only a form of energy. We also have to rid ourselves of the feeling that we must struggle to get it and struggle to keep it. Life without debt can be so freeing. Even large mortgages can be paid off over time.

The main thing is to concentrate on the feeling of freedom from heavy obligations. Without that feeling, we will keep creating the debt over and over again or something else which weighs us down. In the next section, I look at how patterns have held me back in my life. I call this section "Illusions of Grandeur" because, as I look back at these periods in my life, I realize that I was living in an illusion.

Illusions of Grandeur

Those of us caught in the "life is a struggle" mentality often are unconsciously attracted to schemes that appear good on the surface but drain away our finances and leave us in the struggle mode.

The wealth trigram emphasizes the gradual accumulation of wealth through persistence, but many of us get caught up with get-rich schemes that hold the promise of fast money. We are always looking for something which will give us financial freedom and the lifestyle of our dreams. We have to be aware that the only way to get that freedom is to release our own debilitating patterns.

I found that I was losing money over and over again in various investments and I finally was forced to look at what I was doing. When I looked at myself honestly, I realized that I was repeating several self-defeating patterns around money.

I continued my "life is a struggle" mentality by getting involved in businesses which took a lot of energy and time and, under my direction, made very little money. I was wooed first into a clothing store, following someone's advice about it being a profitable business and not checking for myself. I went headlong into it, putting myself into tremendous debt and, not wanting to admit failure, struggled to keep this business alive for 10 years. Borrowing money for this business mortgaged my house completely, as well as took all my salary. I had to work elsewhere to support it. Strangely enough, this business is still operating, owned by my manager who took it over from me and it has been a struggle for her as well.

At the same time, I set up my "I am a victim" mentality by getting involved in land and property investments, using up sizeable savings, and lost all of them. These deals were presented to me by people whom I trusted because they told me what I wanted to hear. I followed their claims of financial freedom without looking at my best interests.

My next big "I am a victim" investment was a 1966 yacht which was supposed to be a charter business with a partner who talked as if he were very interested but eventually pulled out and left me on my own. This business took a great deal of money over 7 years and eventually the boat was donated. As I discuss elsewhere, the boat had a spiritual purpose but, from a financial viewpoint, it was a continuous drain. With this investment, I set up a situation in which I was in the control of workmen and captains whom I would struggle to pay without question, because I knew very little about the running of this 47 foot boat.

If I had taken this lost money and invested it, I would be a multi-millionaire today. Instead of that, I was subconsciously attracted towards investments which were a struggle and drained all my money away. What would make me do that? Believing that money was a struggle and was hard to get, I created a situation that would prove this. I could have created a pleasant life style but because subconsciously, I believed that I should struggle, I created businesses that took a lot of work and kept me fighting for money.

All these investments were very risky and none of them were wise investments such as my parents would have made. Subconsciously, there may have been a rebellion against my parents since they approved of none of these things. I was trying, on another level, to impress them and, on another, prove that I couldn't make it.

Why would I be drawn to such choices? I believe that there are many reasons. The first is that I needed to stay in the struggle mentality. Also, I had several patterns related to fear of success and not deserving money. There was also an issue of putting myself in the control of other people in order to fulfill "the victim mentality." There are always many unconscious processes taking place at one time. When we are engaged in unconscious patterns, hurting ourselves is part of the process. Unconsciously, we are also proving to ourselves that we can't keep money or that we don't deserve to have it.

There are lessons to learn in financial crises. If I had made wise decisions with my money and had made a lot of it, I might not have started to look at myself and develop myself spiritually. There is a spiritual reason behind all our adversity.

Years later, after becoming aware and conscious of my patterns, I met one of the men who had "victimized" me, taking a huge amount of money from me. He had wooed me with talk of big developments which would give me financial freedom.

After he had lost my money and that of others, he had continued to wheel and deal and eventually settled in Spain, afraid to come back and face family and friends. He eventually lost all his money and was brought back by air ambulance after he suffered a stroke.

When I first saw him, after all those years, it was difficult not to feel angry at this man who had walked away with my savings at a very hard time in my life. But with my present understanding, I got beyond the anger and saw a shell of a man who had nothing left in his life. I expected him to say that he was sorry but, instead, I saw a man who felt no remorse and was more upset that he had lost all that was of value in his life. He kept talking about all the money he had had at one time.

I reminded him that he had some kind of lesson to learn from all this and that there must be a reason that he was still alive. Instead of looking at the spiritual significance, this man was lost in the past, still blaming others for his present condition. I left him, feeling glad that I was able to face him without bitterness. Seeing him again reminded me of the shift that had taken place in my life. I finally knew that money, in itself, was not the panacea that I had felt it to be. In fact, unless we have the state of mind first to "be" a certain way, we will never be able to "do" and "have" true abundance. In the next section, I look at how this thinking is a paradigm shift for most of us in our culture.

Be, Do, Have

In our world, we have been taught to go after the things we think we need—the status, the power, the education, and the money. We must seek these things in order to do the things to make us happy. The worldly paradigm emphasizes "having" first, then "doing" in order to "be" happy, fulfilled etc.

For instance, I was taught to seek out education first in order to have the things that would give me the money and the freedom to pursue the things that were meaningful to me. The theory was that education would lead me to jobs that would bring money and possessions and our family would be able to do things that we enjoyed—go to country clubs, travel all over the world, etc. These things would make us happy.

I saw my parents spending so much of their time preoccupied

with investing money in the stock market while my father worked very hard at dentistry to be able to have things—the house, the cars, the clothes etc. What I also saw was a hollowness in their actions.

Even though they were making money, they were always worried about when the stock market would go down. When I started to invest money later in land, my father would tell me that land was a poor investment because the value of it could go down very fast. Looking from a fresh and innocent point of view, I could see that all investments had this problem. Everything controlled by people could go up and down with their whims. It became apparent to me that there was nothing safe about the investments of the world, so there had to be something beyond them to give you security.

If you think doing things depends on having a backup of money or possessions, your security can disappear in a moment. My father would say that I could not or should not do something, like take a trip, until I had enough money to back it up. When I had enough money to be able to do the things that I wanted to do, then I was allowed to be happy.

As I was growing up, I realized that the times that I was happiest did not have much connection with having things. The most content times for me were when I was in a natural setting, just enjoying the surroundings and connecting with nature. As I look at it now, these were probably the times when I was able to connect with my spiritual side. Through nature, we see that there is something beyond ourselves and that there appears to be some divine order in the universe.

When I got married, however, I continued the paradigm that I had been taught, seeking out possessions (the big house, the cars etc.) in order to be able to do things (play tennis, go to expensive restaurants, join a country club, take nice trips etc.) and felt that I should be truly happy. I found that my life, like my parents, was feeling empty. I had the resources to be able to do the things that made me happy. Why was I feeling like this?

I decided to leave my first marriage and go back to school and get more education. Maybe this would increase my happiness. My education has been very helpful in taking me to my chosen work but it, in itself, did not make me happy. I thought that I would try another relationship since my marriage had not brought me happiness, even though we were able to have a great deal of material things.

In my second marriage, I tried to put more emphasis on building the relationship but soon found that we, too, were lost in the search for possessions, thinking that these things would bring happiness. At one time, I had a store, cottage, 2 houses, a condo, an apartment and a yacht. Each of these possessions took a great deal of time and money to maintain. As I had less and less money, I was more and more harassed and pressured. I did not even think about relationships or happiness.

When I lost money on each of these things and lost my full-time employment, I was no longer able to pay for them. My marriage was breaking up because of the pressure. As a result of all this adversity, I started to turn my attention to the message in spiritual writings. I was able to open up to another side of myself that was telling me I was looking in the wrong places for satisfaction.

I started to look back over my possessions and ask myself if they had ever brought me happiness. Other than a temporary pleasure from time to time, the answer was no. What brought me pleasure was to be able to go to my cottage and walk in the woods or swim in the lake or feel the peace of the ocean in my boat. These things could be enjoyed without the possession.

As I started to let go of these possessions and simplify my life, I felt such a release and was able to turn my attention completely to spiritual readings and studying practices like Qigong, T'ai Chi

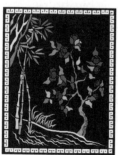

Ch'uan and Feng Shui. These things made me realize that there was a part of me that I had buried for many years in that wild pursuit for things.

I realized that if I could just be a more spiritual, loving and caring person, I could feel the happiness that I was searching for. How could I know that I was more spiritual?

The only way that I could do this was to share it with others. What I was learning made more sense when I explained it to clients and friends and radiated this new feeling to others through my actions.

What we don't realize is that we have to "be" a certain way in order to do the things that are meaningful and then we will "have" the things which are important for us. To be happy, we have to find that happiness inside, the Spirit inside, the connection to the divine and we know that we have it when we share it with others.

We cannot share it in an artificial way. It must be sincere because, when we are sincere, we are coming from the heart. The old phrase "fake it until you make it" is misleading because, when we are insincere, our subconscious knows it and we do not experience true feelings.

When we desire happiness or money or anything else, we need to give up our fear and give to another what we desire for ourselves and miraculously, the same will come to us. We are showing our subconscious mind that we have enough of something to give to another and we convince it that we have it. We set up an energy that will attract to us the things that will take us further on our path. When we can concentrate on feeling good instead of needing something, whatever we need will come to us. Even when we don't have it, we can give it to another. This is hard to do in our world but, as we flow with the universe, we attract abundance and share it with others.

Most of us have reversed the paradigm and we search for our happiness in a better body, better relationships or more possessions. When these things fail us, we become disillusioned and depressed instead of taking the opportunity to concentrate on "being." From our being comes the feeling to do the things that make us happy and, from doing those things, we start to have what we need. When we start to get a sense of who we are, we start to do the things which feel more like our purpose. However, amassing wealth can be part of our purpose. Let us take a closer look at the meaning of wealth.

Wealth

In our society, it may be important to have wealth, but it cannot be our sole reason for existence. We get caught up in the making of money to the exclusion of all else. As well as seeing money as our "living," when we finally start to make excess money, we spend a great amount of time trying to figure out how to invest it and make it grow.

In the long run, we need to ask ourselves why are we living here on earth at this time. Does it make sense that it is just to make money? Even if we do not believe in anything beyond this world, does it make sense that we are here to amass money and then die and leave it?

With the world changing around us, we are still absorbed and preoccupied with how to make money, how to invest it and how to spend it. It reminds me of the depiction of the Titanic when it was going down. The wealthy were so absorbed with what they were doing that they did not recognize that the boat was sinking.

If we put our attention on money alone, we will miss what we are here on earth to do. It is when people have a great deal of money and everything that money can buy that they realize that it alone does not bring them any satisfaction or happiness. What appears to bring people satisfaction is some kind of meaning or purpose to their lives. They then use their money to help others.

Your purpose might be demonstrated in a hobby or in a job. You might be a financier, a stockbroker or a computer analyst but, in doing these things, you feel happy and completed. Often you are directly helping others or you might be providing a needed worldly service. The key is whether you love doing what you are doing. The way of knowing your purpose is by asking yourself if you would be doing this thing, even if you received no money to do it. It is just the way you like to spend your time.

When you take the emphasis off money, you start to concentrate on the joy of what you are doing. If you are not doing what you like to do, you start to spend time looking for things that give you pleasure. You start to look at your relationships and how you can help others. You begin to take satisfaction in simple things, like watching children play or listening to birds sing.

If we do the things we love to do without worrying about how the money will come, it mysteriously starts to come. When we become more aligned to our purpose and we have more idea about how we are going to serve the world, we get ourselves in flow with the universe. There are metaphysical texts that suggest that, in higher levels of consciousness, everything that is needed in the material world can be brought forth from the universe and then returned to a nonmaterial form when it isn't needed anymore. It appears to me that that is how enlightened societies would work. If we focused less on money, we could choose to move on the path of joy instead of a path of struggle.

The Path of Struggle or the Path of Joy

Most of us have learned to walk on the path of struggle, as I have pointed out, and one of the places that it demonstrates itself the most is in the area of finances. Most of us have learned that we need to struggle to get money and struggle to keep it. That is why debt has such an unconscious appeal to us since it takes away most of what we earn and leaves us in that struggle mentality. We can work hard to get money and then struggle to get ahead because we have to pay our creditors.

What is the alternative? Is there indeed a way of living in joy? I believe that there is. We can have fun making money and enjoy abundance. The laws of the universe are such that all of us should be enjoying abundance. Scarcity, however, is something that the world believes in and so we create it everywhere.

How can we create abundance? First, we must clear the subconscious messages which say that we have to suffer and struggle. In order to clear them, we need to bring that consciousness to full awareness. Look at how you feel about money. Do you have fear around it? Do you believe that it is difficult to keep? Do you believe that it is difficult to make?

As we bring forward our true feelings, we acknowledge that these attitudes are holding us back, knowing that we can change them. We connect with that part of us that is holding us back and sometimes relive the feeling of that part. For most of us, it is the child in us who is still living back in early times, learning from parents that money was difficult to get.

In order to really achieve abundance, we need to be able to feel abundant first. Abundance is not synonymous with money. There are many people with money who do not feel abundant. We are not concerned with stockpiling our goods. Instead, we believe that everything we need will flow to us. It is a feeling devoid of worry and fear.

To achieve this feeling of abundance, we should have in our mind the qualities that we think abundance will give us in our life. How do we want to feel as a result of this abundance? For me, I want the feelings of peace, serenity, simplicity and joy.

The point is that I do not need to have money to have these feelings. It is better to create these feelings first. The contradiction is that, if we do not achieve these feelings first, we will not receive them from money. In fact, money can make our life more complex and, in some cases, burdened.

Some people want the feelings of security, but if you do not cultivate these feelings first, the irony is that money will not give them to you. I have seen a lot of people who have a lot of money and who do not feel secure at all. They are always concerned that they are making the wrong investments and that they will lose their money. Also people feel that they will become more powerful with money. Often they feel more powerless because their investments are under the control of others.

We have to remember that neither security nor power comes with money but instead come with our connection to the spiritual power within us. As we connect with that Inner Power, we will be more in touch with joyful living.

As we develop the qualities that we want money to give us, we will start to magnetize the conditions and people around us that will bring the abundance that we want. A place to observe true abundance is in nature. When I am feeling lack or limitation, I always take a walk in nature and try to concentrate on the lessons I can learn there. This area of the bagua is the element of wood which comes from trees.

Teachings of Nature

I have two trees in my garden in South Florida, which have been teaching me about abundance. One is an orange tree and the other is a key lime tree. They demonstrate to me different theories of abundance. The key lime tree always has a few blossoms on it and some fruit and, a couple times a year, has an abundance of fruit. The orange tree has most of its blossoms at once and the fruit is available for at least four months a year.

I believe that these two patterns show us how we can have abundance in our life. In the case of the key lime tree, a little flows to us all the time and then there are certain times when there is more. Sometimes we fare more like the orange tree. We put all our energy into blossoming ideas and projects and the abundance doesn't flow right away. It comes after a time of seemingly no action.

Neither tree is ever dormant. There is always some activity while the blossoms are forming or the fruit is growing. It is the same with us. There is always an idea which will come to fruition at a later time. Even the word fruition reminds us of something coming "to fruit."

As I watch the blossoms on the orange tree, I am entranced by the fact that these little flowers become first the small pea-sized fruit and then the big juicy oranges which we eat. The tree drops several of the small oranges along the way, but there is always an abundance of fruit.

For us, the lesson is that, although we may think of several ideas, some get left along the wayside but many become long-range projects. The main lesson to learn from these trees is that everything is done without effort, as if according to a divine plan. In nature, nothing is forced. It just happens.

When we feel lack, we begin to worry and wonder if anything is ever going to happen to our project. Instead of planting a seed and allowing the natural course of the universe to help us, it is human nature to interfere with the process when we don't see anything happening. We have planted the seed and all we need to do is water it once in a while and leave it on its own. A farmer does not dig into the soil to see if his crops are rooted and growing. Once he has planted the seed, he is confident that the plant will grow.

It is the same process for us when we are starting a new project. Once we have planted the seed we need to let it stay in the ground until it is ready to sprout. It may seem dormant, but there is always some activity taking place. All we need to do is give it energy and we will attract the people and events to help us.

I am reminded of many times in my life when I had some ideas about where I wanted to go but was not sure how to get there. The more I worried about it, the more complicated I made it. A good example of that was how I got the papers to stay in the United States. As I mention elsewhere, many synchronistic events brought me to this country and I didn't even know why I was here. I just let the course of events happen and found myself here. When I decided that I wanted to stay here however, I started to worry about how the process of getting a "green card" was going to take place and tried to orchestrate events. What I did seemed to make matters worse until I thought that I would have to go back to Canada to live.

When I surrendered to the idea of returning to Canada, events started to take place to make it possible for me to stay. I stopped trying hard and simply let events unfold. It is the same with anything in life. If we try too hard, we interfere with the process.

In the past few months, I received another lesson from my key lime tree. In a severe storm, the tree split in three pieces and fell to the ground. The next day I mourned my loss as I surveyed the broken tree with the fruit all over the ground. However, I realized that sometimes these trees can be saved and called a gardener to see what he could do. He was able to put the parts of the broken trunk together and hold them with a rope until they can grow on their own. He had to cut off most of the branches but I notice that the little tree that is left is already starting to blossom again.

This is the hardest lesson for us to learn, the one when we lose everything and have to put together the pieces to start again. Our dreams have disappeared and we think that all is lost. If we stay strong, we will see opportunities coming back slowly - blossom by blossom.

The next section gives you an exercise to attract opportunities, events and people which will bring more abundance into your life.

Becoming Magnetic to What You Want Exercise

We are always attracting people and circumstances to us, whether we know it or not. To be able to attract what we want consciously is the key.

The first thing that you do is get a clear picture of what you want to achieve in your life. More importantly, try to be aware of the essence that you want to have when it comes into being (like a feeling of joy or happiness). Sometimes we decide that we want a specific thing and when it comes to us we do not want it because it does not bring the feelings we wanted.

The concentration should be on being a certain way, not having specific things.

Get the picture very clear of what you want, a clear picture of how you see yourself living.

Concentrate on love for whatever you want to create and, through this love, how you might provide a service for others. The more you see the service of what you have to offer, the more magnetic you become.

After we have fixed an idea in our mind, the next step is to visualize what we want. Our concentration acts as a magnet and brings to us the people and events which help us create our image.

It is better not to discuss what you are doing because you attract the criticism of other people, so keep silent about what you are trying to manifest unless you are with people who will help support your dream.

Before we visualize, we need to have in our mind the feeling or essence of what we desire. As I said before, the more that we concentrate on the service that our creation will render, the more it will be rewarded with money.

The next important component of the visualization is the feeling of having achieved whatever we want. The more real and emotional we make the picture, the more real the circumstances are created in our life. Thoughts energized by emotions attract vibrations which harmonize with what is uppermost in the mind. That is precisely why we need to keep our thoughts happy and harmonious. Keep yourself centered in a feeling of abundance.

It is best to write down your plan concisely in words, again concentrating on the essence or feeling you want to have. Then read it over out loud as many times a day as possible and always before you go to sleep and again when you wake up in the morning. These two times are the times when you reach the subconscious mind the easiest and you are most suggestible.

Affirmations

I have joy and peace in my life.
I love my work and provide a service for others doing it.
I attract events and people into my life which bring me abundance.
Abundance comes to me easily and effortlessly

FENG SHUI FOR YOUR ENVIRONMENT

This is your area of fortunate blessings of all kinds. The element is wood. The following are good is this area:

- Anything that makes you feel abundant
- The colors red, purple, gold and silver
- An arrangement of coins
- A water fountain, symbolizing abundance flowing
- A plant growing upward, symbolizing growth

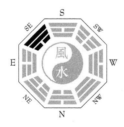

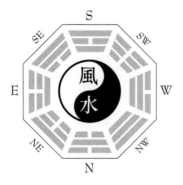

CHAPTER 5

T'ai Chi

T'ai Chi

The center of the bagua is the T'ai Chi, represented by the familiar symbol of Yin and Yang, each containing a seed of the other. T'ai Chi means supreme ultimate, or perfect balance of Yin and Yang, what the Chinese refer to as the masculine and feminine principles of life. Yin is the dark, passive, yielding, soft, pliant side of life, and yang is the light, active, aggressive, hard side of life. It is not good to be too much of one or the other but the best is to have both in balance. This symbol also represents the circular nature of the cycle of life, the seasons and the compass directions.

The T'ai Chi symbol is in the center of the bagua (and your house) representing the harmony achieved when all areas of our life are in order. It relates to health—not just absence of sickness—but living free and unburdened. It refers to the balance achieved when we are living our purpose, having loving partnerships, respecting our elders, having good fortune in our everyday life, helping others and being helped by others, sharing ourselves through our creative endeavors and our progeny, taking time to contemplate our essence and being known as a person of integrity and mastery. It is the center where we stay grounded and focused, our feet firmly planted on the earth; the element of this area of the bagua. The colors here are shades of earth.

In this area, we look at my experience with the practice of T'ai Chi Ch'uan, the lessons that I learned from it, and living in harmony with the natural elements.

The Lessons of T'ai Chi Ch'uan

I was first introduced to T'ai Chi Ch'uan in Toronto, Canada where I was living at the time. I had seen the Chinese people out in parks in both Toronto and Vancouver doing that slow, balletic movement but never knew what it was. At the time of my study of Chinese students, I discovered that the students who practiced this type of movement were able to handle their stress better.

It was just after that period that I, too, discovered the power of these practices. As I mentioned in the introduction, I was, at that time, living a very stressful life working several jobs and taking care of two teenage sons as a single mother. I had received an injury after strenuous exercise, my form of relaxation at that time. Because of this injury, I was introduced to acupuncture and then T'ai Chi Ch'uan, practices that healed my back pain. The acupuncturist taught me that energy flows through pathways of the body and that it can be stimulated by placing needles at certain points on this pathway. She told me that I could induce the flow of energy myself through the practices of T'ai Chi Ch'uan and Qigong.

My first experience with T'ai Chi Ch'uan was under the tutelage of a fellow university adjunct professor who was fascinated by the health benefits that she had witnessed in people studying with a Taoist monk who had settled in Toronto. She had seen miraculous changes in arthritis, multiple sclerosis, and even cancer. She was very apologetic about her own skill, recognizing that it took many years to become a master in this discipline. What I did learn from her was the calmness and peacefulness of these movements.

Over the years, I have studied various forms of Qigong and T'ai Chi Ch'uan under many masters, both Chinese and Western, and have realized that there are certain principles that underlie all forms. What interests me is how these principles apply, not only to the movement, but to our lives in general. All of them are lessons also apparent in the Feng Shui bagua.

Principle 1: Release the blocks

T'ai Chi Ch'uan has been used for centuries in China to promote health and longevity. It is a slow, flowing movement that has a great effect on your body. T'ai Chi Ch'uan is a form of Qigong which means working with energy.

This energy, called Qi, life force energy, is flowing through everything and keeping you alive. In the body, Qi flows through meridian channels and, when flowing freely, helps eliminate illness. The Chinese believe that blocks in these channels are related to disease. Similar to how an acupuncturist puts needles into your body to stimulate the free flow of energy, Feng Shui makes changes in your environment to enhance the flow of energy. The movement of Qigong and T'ai Chi Ch'uan is like natural acupuncture, circulating the energy in the body through movement and intention.

Where does this energy come from? The Taoist practices believe it is formed from the original energy of our parents and is the essence of what we eat and breathe but, more than that, we are also linked with universal force energy. When we are conscious of this link, we move with the flow of life, not against it, and can accomplish anything.

Principle 2: Action is not always necessary

The movements of T'ai Chi are like a metaphor of how to live life. The Wu Chi stance, the T'ai Chi form's opening and closing positions of emptiness, is the place where the potential movement has not begun yet or has ended. It is that very necessary state between non-action and action. In our worldly actions, it is when we stand still for a minute, reassess and choose our next action. As we stand in this position in full awareness, we get in touch with the blockages in our body. We become aware of pain in certain places and we know that these are emotional blocks that have solidified in our body over time. In our life, this time of non-action helps us get in touch with intuition, guidance or inspiration to know what is the next step on our path. If we stay still and get in touch with inner strength, we will know how to circumvent obstacles.

Principle 3: We cannot judge a situation

We learn to empty our mind of all thoughts which intrude upon us. By concentrating on the slow movement and on our breath, we find that disturbing thoughts, which might have been there at one time, have disappeared from our mind. Over time, in these practices, we learn not to judge our emotions. We will feel the intensity of them but not for long and will be able to see, as in the T'ai Chi symbol, that there is always the seed of opportunity in all situations that we perceive as a problem.

Principle 4: Life is a circle

To achieve harmony is the main aim of Taoist practices. Realizing that there is this dual quality of all things means recognizing that in all perceived harmful situations, there is the seed of the opposite quality. If you look at the Yin/Yang symbol, you will see that each part flows into the other, each is half of the same whole and each contains a seed of the other. In fact, the whole image represents a circle or a sphere which represents the harmonious movement of life. As you watch T'ai Chi Ch'uan as a form, you will observe the circular motion of all the movements and how many of them, if watched closely, look like the T'ai Chi symbol. Just like the movement of T'ai Chi, the soft changes into the hard and vice versa or you are moving from one state to the other. In the same way, life is moving in a dynamic and circular motion. Whatever we send out returns to us.

Principle 5: Cultivate a quiet mind

The ultimate aim of Taoist practices, however, is to feel our emotions but to not let them take hold—to cultivate a quiet mind. The practices of Qigong and T'ai Chi Ch'uan train us to move slowly and consciously, not getting caught up in our thoughts, in touch with any part of the body that feels painful. Instead of ignoring it or taking a pill to get rid of it, we hear its cry for help and realize that this is a part of us where our emotions are blocked. The tensions that we feel in our body have been built up for years by our reaction to the stresses around us. This movement helps us release these old blockages.

When our mind is quiet, we can hear the messages that our body is giving us. We can get impressions from our senses, emotions and gut feelings. We become mindful of everything around us and know its place in our life. From the perspective of a quiet mind, we can access guidance and move forward on our path, circumventing obstacles.

Principle 6: Stay in full awareness

Each movement in T'ai Chi is done in full awareness. As we move slowly, effortlessly, gracefully, we are aware only of the movement, nothing else. It is a good example of living life in the present moment, concentrating only on what is happening in each instant.

Principle 7: Know when to go forward and when to Retreat

What we are learning in the movement and philosophy of Taoist T'ai Chi Ch'uan are other ways of looking at things demonstrated in the movement. One of the major ideas in T'ai Chi Ch'uan is the movement between Yin and Yang. In the practice of T'ai Chi Ch'uan, we alternate between these two positions. At times, we have one part of our body in a Yang position and another is in a

Yin position. What this demonstrates in life is the flow between these two positions.

The movement is from full to emptiness, from insubstantial to substantial, from a forward movement to a backward movement. In life, we have to know when to move forward and when to retreat. We must become aware that the retreat can come right after an aggressive stance. There is a time to be active and a time to be passive. As we live in full awareness, we know that the opposite effect is just behind. When we feel sadness, we know that joy is very close behind.

Principle 8: Remain detached

What we seek is balance and not being attached to either state. As we adopt this philosophy, we search for this place of balance where we can easily move from one state to the other and not feel stuck in either. We feel harmony in all things and, when harmony deserts us for a while, we don't get upset because we know that it will return.

Sometimes we have to be more active, but often, yielding is the best response. As we flow between these two positions, we stay in the knowledge that there is always another perspective, that things are not as they seem and there is a more spiritual way to view any event. T'ai Chi Ch'uan is a Taoist martial art which teaches us to go with the flow and not oppose the opponent's force. We deflect the energy and return it.

Principle 9: Live in the Present

In T'ai Chi Ch'uan, we lose our focus if we anticipate the next position before we move into it. In life, we often live in the future instead of the present so we are never fully in the moment. To concentrate fully on each movement, even though it is a flow of motion, teaches us to stay with our concentration fixed in the present, if only for a second. It gets us in the practice of being fully in the moment and the more we do it, the more often we can stay in the present for a longer period of time.

Principle 10: Cultivate the Mind/Body/Spirit

The idea is to keep our bodies relaxed during this movement and let the mind be at peace. It is what is called mindfulness movement. As we focus only on our movements, we allow our mind to be free of thoughts. As we calm the mind and relax the body, we allow ourselves to become calm and detached, permeating this feeling into our outer world. At the same time, our slow, deep breaths bring harmony to our mind and body. While Westerners would say that the purpose of Qigong is to improve health, the Chinese would say that it is to cultivate the three treasures—the energy found in the three centers, the upper center (shen), the heart center (qi) or the lower center (jing) or, as we would think of it, the body, mind and spirit. Some of the higher level Qigong cultivation practices are based on a very spiritual view of the world. One major goal of all Qigong is greater harmony inside and outside. To create more harmony, we need to live within the principles of the Tao. One of those principles is to balance the polarities, the Yin and the Yang.

What We Resist Persists

To achieve balance, we need to work at unifying, instead of splitting off or resisting one side. One of the major polarities that we deal with is the male and female. The male is viewed as the analytical way of seeing things, the wish to cut things into pieces, to label things, to measure things and to see them in linear form, one thing following another in logical order. The male intellect dis-

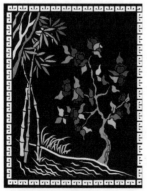

sects and analyzes and does not often see things as a whole. The female energy tends to look at things as a whole, sees life as a process, feels instead of thinks, trusts intuition and yields instead of attacks. What we need to do is embrace these two energies inside of us and allow ourselves to be comfortable with both.

In order to succeed in our male-oriented society, many females have taken on a male way of viewing things. If both males and females would nurture and respect the intuitive, as well as the logical and rational, way of seeing things, they would have the power of both sides. If, as well, we can honor the different aspects of being both male and female, we can respect each other and give each other power.

As with the differences between male and female, we tend to view everything in terms of polarities. We are either sad or happy. We want to get rid of the one side in order to reach the other. When we are sad, we find that a bad place to be and want to achieve the opposite state which is happiness. But as long as we deny the importance of the one side to get to the other, we are always bouncing back and forth between the two. Instead of resisting sadness, if we were to accept it and understand its lesson, we would soon reach equilibrium.

The contradiction about trying to get away from something is that when we resist it, it sticks to us even harder. This is true whether it be a job, a relationship or an event in life. The more we dwell on it, particularly in a negative manner, the more we hold it to us.

We need to adopt a stance of openness and yielding, important qualities of the Tao. In order to get there, we have to be in a position of balance ourselves. If we are obsessed with something, it is sapping all our power and we are not able to find our center.

Often I have situations with people whom I allow to take me off center. I want to reduce involvement with these people but I find the process of removing myself takes all my energy. I find myself thinking about it, talking to others about it, and not finding a solution.

From my Eastern practices, I know that the way to resolve any situation is to stand firm and centered and allow it to take care of itself. It is like the model of a tree with its roots firmly in the ground, bending to the storms of change but not becoming uprooted.

Wu Chi meditation is like that. You stand in an upright position with your hands hanging loosely by your side. Your feet are parallel, shoulder-width apart and your knees and hip joints are loosely relaxed. Your goal is to stay relaxed and release parts of your body. As you stand this way, you discover habitual ways that you have held your body, sometimes with muscles tight and chest puffed up or shoulders sagging. Your first step is to find your balance and sometimes you find that you are compensating for an unbalanced feeling by tightening muscles. You first learn to relax your mind and then your body.

As you stand for longer periods you learn to relax your body, opening your muscles, joints and tendons. By patiently allowing your body to change, your joints will start to open and your body will start to become naturally aligned.

In the same way, we learn to come to balance in situations and relationships in our lives. When we tense up and resist, we become obsessed with the situation and cannot see the forest for the trees. In relationships, we dwell on our expectations of others or of ourselves and cannot get a clear, unbiased picture.

When we have expectations of situations or of people, we can never relax because we are watching everything so carefully to see if everything is going according to how we want it to go. We have given up our power because we can't be happy or satisfied until something outside our control changes. All our energy is used up trying to alter a situation or relationship and we are completely off balance.

How can we stay balanced around unbalanced situations? The key is to stay centered in our mind and body. If we let go and search only for balance in ourselves, we discover our blocks. When I start to obsess about anything, I bring my attention back to my body and notice what those obsessions are doing to it physically. As I mentioned before, these unresolved emotions become blocks in our body. As I stand and try to relax through the stiffness and soreness, I think of all the unfinished situations that I have been holding onto. As I start to let go physically, I start to let go mentally.

The only way I can control a situation is by controlling my own feelings about it. When I pit my will against another, I am setting up a situation that I cannot control and that will put me off center.

When we take a stance of balance, we are open to anything that happens but we are not put off center by it. We are what is called self-referred; that is, we know that our power is inside and not from anything around us. It is to know that we have a divine purpose and that everything that comes to us is there for a reason. We have only to wait in a balanced way to find the true meaning and not to get caught up by the ups and downs.

This principle is demonstrated in the ancient story of the farmer who had two things that he truly valued, his son and a horse. One day his horse disappeared and he was in the depths of despair. When the horse reappeared with a wonderful mare, he was very happy. His son rode the new horse and fell and broke his leg and the farmer was again in the depths of despair. However, a war broke out and all the young men were taken off to war except his son who could not go because of his disability. Again the farmer was very happy. This story shows a man who is completely controlled by outside events. The farmer's emotions went up and down according to what was happening in his life. If he had remained calm and detached, he would have known that there was an overall purpose to what was happening, even if he could not figure it out at the moment.

If we wait in a balanced way, we will see over time the significance of events in our lives. Just as in that story, something that appears to be a dire circumstance at the time may have a positive outcome. We cannot judge. When we create balance in our own life, we will start to attract balance around us. Chaos and confusion no longer serve us and we will move towards things that are peaceful and more harmonious. One of the places where we are reminded of this state is in nature.

Nature

I sit here by the beach in Florida, thinking that I do not get here as much as I need to. I live close by but rarely get here. It is a sad commentary on our lives that we have beautiful natural surroundings about us but we never see them. I learned, as a child, that being in nature was very balancing. Almost every weekend our family would take walks in a park or in the woods.

As a teenager, I did not want to go to summer camp in northern Ontario but when I got there, I was wooed by the beauty of the lakes and trees. I remember sitting on those sturdy rocks looking over the lake, feeling completely at peace. Some of my happiest memories as a child were those experiences in a natural surrounding.

It is a known fact that nature gives you positive energy which soothes you. It also lets you take another view of a problem that may be consuming you. If you go into a natural surrounding and sit with something that is bothering you, after a while you start to get calm and you allow the universe to speak to you.

We are always rushing and running around, distracted by the events and problems in our lives. The spiritual literature tells us that answers to all our problems are there for our asking, if we would allow them to come. So often we focus on the problem, not ever seeing beyond it to the solution. Nature provides some of these answers for us.

We watch trees firmly rooted in the ground. When a storm comes, they may toss and sway but they do not lose their roots. When man does not interfere with it, each part of nature has its place and it operates in complete harmony. When the birds get up in the morning, they do not worry about how they are going to live through the day. They have faith that they will find the food they need and they sing.

Feng Shui emerged from the desire to live in harmony with nature. The ancients observed their surroundings and saw where the land was more prosperous and noticed that there was more abundant energy there. They set up their structures to be in harmony with this abundant energy. They also set up their villages or towns surrounded by hills or mountains which protected them from adverse weather. One of the most tranquil settings is like an armchair where there is a hill behind, like the back of a chair and a peaceful view of water in front.

How can we live more in harmony with nature? One way is

to set aside at least one time a day to sit quietly in nature, even if it is a city park. In Hong Kong, I was able to find perfect peace in a city park surrounded by tall buildings and business people running by. Many people were there, enjoying their morning physical movement, oblivious to the distractions around them.

When you get up in the morning, try to see how many birds you can hear. As you sit in nature, sit quietly and try to empty your mind from its usual chatter. As you transcend your usual thoughts and concentrate on just what is around you, you will see that you will be transported into another world, one where nothing matters in the same way, one where you know there will be answers to questions even if you don't know what they are.

Nature gives us the assurance to know that we are here for a space in time and that our life is not as it seems. The more you sit there, the more you realize that there is something which is much bigger than you, some kind of divine plan of which you are a part. What is that part? If you contemplate the stillness, you will start to get some sense of it. Most of the time you are too busy to notice.

A few years ago I bought a cottage in northern Ontario. We used to get up early in the morning to go up there and I would wake up with anticipation of the peace I would feel as we got to the highway where the lakes were all in view. I looked forward to arriving in the beautiful wooded surroundings and even having a dip in the wonderful velvet water of the lake.

I would arrive there carrying all my bills and my course preparations, having my mind clogged with all the problems of my various responsibilities. If I did all this work back home, I would feel overwhelmed and frightened; the more I worked, the worse it became. When I sat in the beauty of nature, however, I would let the peace come over me and I would do the work with one part of my mind on it and the other on my surroundings. I would often sit out on a porch overlooking the lake with the beautiful big pines full of birds and animals and I would allow my creativity to guide me. When I did not obsess about my work, it would get done in due course and without much effort.

I would usually arrive at the cottage late on a Saturday evening after being in my clothing store all day and come back early Monday morning in time to teach or do my administrative work, ready to handle a full week of work. I survived that period of my life because of that brief stay in nature every weekend, even in the dead of winter. Even if the drive was difficult, I would still feel that peace come over me as we hit the more quiet part of the highway.

The most important part of all this is to be able to translate the peace that you feel around you into peace inside of you. The peace that you get in nature helps you feel yourself part of it, to feel at one with it.

As you sit quietly and let your thoughts subside, you start to transcend reality. The thoughts and problems that were consuming you start to lose their importance. The next exercise is one that you can use to help you get to this peaceful state.

Rooting Exercise

There is a practice in T'ai Chi and Qigong, in fact in most martial arts, called rooting. If you watch practitioners, you will see how their movement is low to the ground. It is important to feel rooted like a tree because we feel the stability of the earth beneath us as we absorb energy from it. Also, the center of gravity of our bodies is in the Tan Tien (at the navel or slightly below) and, if we concentrate our energy there, it is hard to be off balance. As we finish these practices, we bring our attention to this place in order to keep the energy stored there. It is the energetic pressure of emotions held in the upper torso that causes heart attacks and other problems originating in the chest.

In the process of rooting, we put our attention into the ground and send down imaginary roots into the ground. Through these roots, we can send our burdens and problems and access healing energy from the ground. The Taoists believe that the earth can recycle destructive energy into positive. Also, the earth is vibrating at a healing rhythm which we can use to heal ourselves. They also believe that we access energy from the universe through the crown of our head and, in fact, as we stand in a balanced position, we become a channel between heaven and earth.

As we go through life, we are often buffeted by events that are happening to us and we allow them to put us off balance. We need to imagine that we are like a tree that bends and sways in a storm but does not become uprooted. I will share with you an exercise simplified from one I learned from a T'ai Chi master, Michael Andron.

- Still your mind by taking some slow, deep breaths.

- Imagine a little seed of light vibrating in your head. Visualize it moving slowly from your head down to your lower center (Tan Tien).

- Feel this center radiating out energy, attuning the whole body to its vibration.

- Imagine two laser beams of light going from your center down each leg, connecting you to the earth's center. Feel yourself linked to the energy of the earth.

- With these roots in place, when you exhale, send your worries, burdens and destructive emotions into the ground to be recycled. When you inhale, draw up healing energy from the earth.

This process can be used any time you feel yourself tossed off balance by events and people. It gives you instant energy as well as a sense of release of problems. It helps you cultivate a quiet mind so that you can get in touch with a sense of peace and, from this space, come up with any decisions that are to be made. You may also imagine your connection with the universe like a cord that extends into the heavens, like a thread attached to the crown of your head.

When we feel these connections, we feel enormous support from the universe around us. We realize that we do not need to handle our problems alone. If we stay silent and peaceful, we can connect with a healing vibration.

Affirmations

I am calm, centered and stable.

I send my burdens into the ground to be recycled.

I am a channel between heaven and earth.

I access healing energy from the universe.

Feng Shui for Your Environment

This is the center of your house and the emphasis here is on things that bring you health and balance. Some examples of these are:

- Healthy plants and flowers
- The T'ai Chi symbol
- Earth tones
- Fresh fruit or artificial fruit
- A skylight or an open area

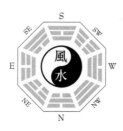

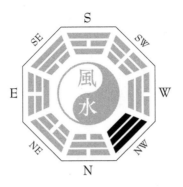

CHAPTER 6
Helpful People

Helpful People Trigram

This trigram, "ch'ien," has three yang lines representing the archetypal father, the leader, the patriarch, heaven and sky. It is the element of big metal, the color of grey, and deals with helpful people and travel. It is on the Northwest corner of your house. This is the trigram of strength and power and looks at both where you take your strength from, as well as how you give strength and power to others. It represents all the people that have been helpful to you, as well as how you have been helpful to people. On the bagua, it is across from wealth and the two are very related. To achieve consistent wealth and abundance in your life, you will need the help of others, as well as to be helpful to others. You can also help people with your abundance.

Travel is part of how you develop your understanding of the world around you, as well as how you impart this understanding to others. In this section, I will look at what I have learned from my travel to Hong Kong, how some of the cultural principles of the Chinese have meaning for us and what we can learn from them. I will also look at how mentors can strengthen your view of yourself, as well as how you can help others find strength. Also, through the power of synchronicity, you can learn to be your own mentor.

Hong Kong

We can learn a lot from travel. All places in the world have information for us to learn. We are attracted to those places that have the strongest message for us. For me, because of my research and many contacts, I had been attempting to go to Hong Kong for many years. Strangely enough, I arrived after the takeover from China. After years of worrying about what might happen after the takeover, Hong Kong seems, on the surface, to be stable and prosperous.

It is modern, glamorous, fast-paced, Western. It exemplifies the many faces of China. It is wildly commercial, bustling and noisy but, under all the material glitz, there is a pulse and undercurrent which is ancient.

The people, like all the Hong Kong Chinese whom I have met in Canada and the United States, are friendly and polite but there is also an underlying discipline in the society that I don't feel in North America. Although there is crime like in all other cities, I sense a feeling of community that we have lost. Especially since they live in confined spaces in Hong Kong, there is an understanding that we need to live in a group or community to survive. I remember when I interviewed students from Hong Kong, I marveled at their commitment to carrying out their obligations to their family to the point of denying their own wishes.

North American culture believes so much in individuality that we neglect the whole. We often deny that we are part of a whole but, for the whole to survive, we must support one another. We must learn to find harmony in our groups. When we learn to have harmony in our relationships and with those around us, we will have harmony on a larger scale, in the world.

The Chinese have an interpersonal concept called "saving face." I learned about this concept when I was doing my study on Chinese students in the early 1980's. It is a way of preserving harmony between people by not exposing your own or another person's weaknesses. I am learning about this concept anew while doing business with the Chinese. There are certain things in which I would like to have more clarity, and in my North American way, I would like to lay everything on the line. I find that difficult to do with the Chinese because, on the surface, everything appears to be fine. I have to find very subtle ways of showing them what I want to change without disturbing our long-term relationship. I find doing business is a combination of binding contracts and building relationships, a balancing act which must be done with great finesse.

What do we have to learn from this concept? If we tried to promote harmony in our relationships and through our community, not exposing others' weaknesses, how would this work? We have been taught to value individuality above all. I do believe, as I said before, that we need to know ourselves first in order to really give to others. What we forget is that, as we develop ourselves, we have more to contribute to the community.

There is another concept in T'ai Chi called Push Hands, a sparring practice in which two people take turns pushing one another. The purpose of this practice, in martial arts terms, is to sense the energy of another to know when to push them off balance. What we can learn by doing this exercise is to work with the flow, understand it, and move with it.

In this practice you understand the opposing force but, more importantly, you understand yourself. The more calm and relaxed you are, the more you can flow with the movement, not resist it. As you continue to do the practice, you develop a feeling of your own strengths and weaknesses, as well as of those of your opponent. To use this model for an interpersonal interaction, you can learn how to work around the weaknesses and emphasize the strengths of yourself and the other people around you. This skill is necessary for helping people, the theme of this area of the bagua. You can learn how to remain centered and calm and, understanding the bigger picture, learn to move with resistance instead of being upset by it.

It seems to me that the solution is to really desire harmony at all costs. As a family mediator, I have seen couples trying to reach a settlement but the underlying motivation is to hurt the other person. The issues they are fighting about, usually children and money, are not the real issues. Usually one or both are really angry and want to get back at the other person, so the children are used as pawns. As I pointed out before, many unresolved issues from childhood surface in relationships and the interaction which is taking place is usually highlighting the early dysfunction, not what is presently going on. When the relationship breaks up, the dysfunctional behavior escalates.

How do we get to that real spirit of cooperation instead of the dysfunction? The answer is to know ourselves as spiritual beings with a purpose here on earth. It is to understand that we are here surrounded by our family of Spirit. I believe that the people who are with us are here because we have agreed to come into this life-time to give lessons to one another. Our life is a journey of discovery and everything that happens to us is giving us a message that we can either learn from or ignore.

When friction happens in our families or communities, it is usually showing us some deeper messages that need to be resolved.

Our strength comes from the knowing that we are all divine beings, that we are all part of a divine plan and that we all have a purpose here on earth. There can be no competition because we all have our place here. With that perspective, it is easy to create a community because we know that we all have a purpose and that we need to support each other's purpose.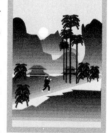

Can you imagine such an enlightened society in which everybody honors everybody else and supports whatever that person does? Unfortunately, our world is still far away from this ideal society, but I believe that we are moving into this under-standing slowly. Even though this type of living does not often exist in Chinese society either, I still detect a deep-seated knowl-edge about living in harmony as a community.

We can only change the society by changing ourselves little by little. As we look around, let us try to see people differently. When we observe people's behavior and see beyond it, we see them as spiritual beings, even though they are not aware of it. As we are truly forgiving, we will start to feel a release of tension as we give up expectations and judgments.

True community exists when we accept all parts of ourselves and then all parts of others. We allow each of us to find our pur-pose and we support each other in this purpose. One way that we can start to do this in our own lives is to mentor ourselves and those around us in this enlightened way.

Mentors

Who has helped you get where you are today? There are always people in our life who influence us along our path. These people may be around for many years or they may appear for a short time just to help us to the next step.

As I look back, there was always someone around to help me see myself differently. As I mentioned, I was a very shy, insecure child who did not believe that I had anything to offer. My mother had a brother who was rough and ready, a sports enthu-siast, who used to come and visit quite often when he finally moved closer to where we lived. He took a special interest in me and called me "the grand dame," a French endearment he learned from French Canada where he had spent most of his life. He seemed to think that I had some kind of flair and, when he was around, I would dress in clothing that gave me a different look, even wearing unique hats.

He had a summer cottage close by and we used to visit there a lot. That was where I first experienced my love of the water and boats and probably had a lot to do with the eventual purchase of the yacht that got me to Florida.

In addition to helping me identify some of my interests, his place was to make me feel special when I did not feel that way generally. He died when I was at university but he had already played a big part in my life.

When I was in school as a child, I had a series of perplexing teachers who insisted on discipline at all costs. The old model "children should be seen and not heard" was very much in place. I was disciplined many times for talking in class and felt afraid and unmotivated most of the time.

School became an ordeal to be endured, a place where you could not be yourself, where you were punished for doing anything natural (like moving and talking) and could be shamed unmercifully at any time.

In Grade 5, I had a male teacher who turned my school career around. He was good looking, young, nice, fun, and, most of all, he was respectful to all the children in the room. Instead of putting us down, he believed that we could do anything. He encouraged us to produce at our highest level and, because he believed we could, we did. It was at this point that my grades started to turn around. I began to see school as something that I could enjoy instead of endure. I started to take an interest in learning for its own sake.

I also started to believe in myself, that I had something to offer instead of feeling that I was no good, the feeling that I received from other teachers. At this age, our feelings about ourselves are very much influenced by the people around us. When a teacher tells you that you will not amount to anything, you tend to believe it. When I was exposed to teachers who believed in me, it made such a difference.

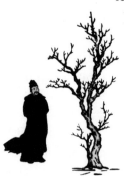

There were at least two in high school. One was a math teacher who was also the coach of the football team when I was a cheerleader. I saw him not long ago when visiting my mother in my hometown. He remembered me, saying that he knew that I would excel at something and leave the crowd behind. He was not surprised that I was living in another country and doing what he considered such interesting work. Perhaps, if he had not been there, in a quiet, encouraging way, I might not have had the courage to take such steps at a later date.

Much later, when I was doing my Ph.D. research, I had two professors who believed my work was important. They were very involved in studying different aspects of the Chinese culture and were glad to support me. They were extremely encouraging about my work and the significance of it, which made me feel that I was doing something worthwhile.

What did these people have in common? They were genuinely interested in who I was as a person and what I wanted to achieve. They urged me to do what I wanted to do and had only support and encouragement, not advice (unless I requested it). They were supportive of the process of discovery and could clarify my confusion when things were not clear for me. They never were opinionated or offered unwarranted suggestions.

The true mentor is there in an unobtrusive way: to clarify, assist, and encourage. Never does the mentor take your lesson away from you. They are there when the going gets tough, as a supporter, not to tell you how to do anything. They can share from their wealth of experience but cannot tell you how to proceed because they trust that only you know how to do this.

The main quality of a mentor, I believe, is to see people at their highest level, to see them in a way that they are unable to see themselves. From a spiritual point of view, it is to focus on the higher self instead of the personality. From the worldly view, it is to concentrate on the strengths of the person instead of the weaknesses.

It is to be completely non-judgmental of the person's behavior. This is often hard to do when we see that they are doing something that we would never do. The goal is to try to understand what they are doing from their perspective, to have empathy or to walk in their shoes for a while. We cannot judge their behavior but we can help them see what they are doing and the implications of that behavior. When someone from the outside points out something to me in a loving way, I am much more open to take a look at it.

The other quality that is important is to motivate and inspire, to point out the larger picture of what is available. I have a mentor today, and he plays an even more spiritual role. He helps to take my problems from the mundane to the spiritual, to see things from a broader perspective. He helps me not to get caught in my own web. He offers philosophy, quotes from higher minds, and different ways of looking at things. He helps me stretch my mind beyond the usual way of looking at things by helping me distinguish the forest from the trees.

How can we be truly helpful to people? We cannot tell anyone how to live their life because we don't know what their path is. We can only point out a broader picture. How can we be more helpful to ourselves? We can be our own mentors as well. Through the process of synchronicity, we are receiving guidance and support from the universe but often we are not open to hear it. The next section helps you be aware of synchronicity in your own life.

Synchronicity

C.G. Jung coined the word "synchronicity" in the foreword of the 1949 English translation of the I Ching by Wilhem and Baynes. He wrote that what we in the West consider random chance, the ancient Chinese regard as a significant event. The I Ching is based on the belief that what we see in the world, at any given time, is a reflection of the underlying reality in which all things are connected and always in a continuous process of change. This philosophy believes that everything that is occurring everywhere is part of the now and nothing exists outside of it.

The I Ching was used as a divination tool for centuries. You ask a question, throw coins to form a pattern of changing trigrams and look up the meaning of the resulting hexagram to receive guidance on a situation.

Synchronicity is a type of divination that gives us answers to sometimes unanswered questions. As we move around in our daily life, we are receiving messages in quite unusual ways, often in the unexplained coincidences that occur. You have probably had an experience in your life when you have been thinking about someone and you see him shortly afterwards, or you hear something on the radio or even read something in a newspaper, which gives you a solution to a problem.

These things can happen all the time, but most of us live our lives without awareness, moving from place to place, without even noticing what is going on around us. We have our plans and our projects and we concentrate on them to the point of fixation. There are synchronistic events occurring everywhere around us at all times but we are not open to them. The answers are always around us but we must be open to receive them.

How do you stay in the spirit of openness when you are bombarded at every given moment by things that need to be done and take all your attention? One of the ways is to remind yourself, at least once an hour, that the world is not as it seems and that the answer you are looking for might be right here, if you would be mindful of the moment. When you are engrossed in something which is especially stressful, try to pull out of it, for even a second, and see what kind of answers might be right around you. If you have any meaningful books, even the Bible, *Tao Te Ching* or another spiritual work, open it up randomly and read what it says. You will see how it connects to your circumstances at that time.

When we work with this knowledge that the answer is always available, we move effortlessly and things seem to open up for us. We move when things flow for us and we stop when things are not flowing. We look for the "synchronicity" in all situations. If we are always busy and preoccupied, we do not see the synchronicity because we are not aware of what is going on around us. It is only in the non-active state that we are able to be aware of these messages.

Sometimes it is a chain of synchronistic messages that we receive that changes our life at a very deep level. For example, in my life, I changed my location, my occupation and my lifestyle because of a boat. On a trip to Florida and the Bahamas, my husband and I met a man who was looking for a partner to do dinner cruises. We were always looking for business opportunities so that we would not be dependent on full time jobs. I had just left the university and vowed not to be caught up in the politics of this kind of organization again. In Florida, I found a large yacht that looked like it would be a good boat for this purpose. It was in an auction sale and we put in a high bid and got it. I did not have the money but I soon went home and arranged mortgages and loans to pay for it. The acquisition of the boat flowed, but I realized later that the boat was not for the purpose I thought.

The partner disappeared and left us with a 47-foot boat that neither of us knew much about. The constant maintenance made it impossible to take it to the Bahamas to use for dinner cruises, but the boat also brought me down to Florida to look after it frequently. I still thought that I would be living in Canada.

While in Florida, on one of these supervising trips, while walking my dog, I ran into a woman with whom I became friendly, and we went to lunch and a bookstore. She highly recommended two books on past-life regression which I read with great interest. They stimulated my interest in hypnosis. When I tried to find this woman later, I couldn't locate her. It was as if she were an angel who had appeared in my life in order to guide me to my next step.

It was through hypnosis that I found my connections in Florida. I met people with whom I conducted workshops and, through a hypnosis course I took, I got connected to a school where I taught and eventually got my "green card."

It was through hypnosis that I started to become really interested in the mind-body connection and linked it to the Eastern practices that I was doing already. As you see, it is a chain of events that make no sense at the time that often can take you in another direction. When I was action-oriented or goal-driven, I would start to push against the flow and many things would come up and make progress very difficult.

When I would stop and reflect and go with the flow, I found that I might not be aware of where I was to end up but I would be attentive and move when it felt right. Now that I look back, the things that were effortless were the things that were most important and each one took me further on my course. Another thing that happened effortlessly was the donating of my boat to a childrens' organization. While I was struggling to sell my boat, an organization asked me to donate it for childrens' programs. Since I had lost so much money on it, I needed to get a certain price. Since that was not happening, I started to entertain the idea of donating it, since I liked what this organization was doing. Even though it made no sense economically, it was because of that donation that I started to do childrens' programs and am now becoming more involved in working with children.

The synchronicity of meeting a man who talked about boats, finding a boat, paying for the boat and being brought down to Florida changed the course of my life. None of it made any sense and, if anyone had told me ten years ago that I would be living in South Florida, I would have said that they were crazy.

We have to be prepared to move with events and let them take us sometimes to unexpected places. These events might not be like anything we have anticipated beforehand. In the next exercise, be aware of how this might have happened already in your own life. Also take time to reflect on what qualities you would like to enhance, making you a successful mentor to yourself and others.

Attracting Helpful People into Your Life

Think about unexpected events in your life. How have they changed the course of events for you? Think about important things in your life. How did they come about?

Think about a challenge in your life now. Open a book at random and see how what you read might give you some new insight. Be open to messages around you. They might come in someone else's words or behavior you observe.

Think about people in your life who have really made a difference. List some of the qualities that inspired and motivated you (such as seeing your better qualities, not judging etc.)

Think about times in your life when you have done the same for others. There have probably been many times when you have inspired and motivated others. List the qualities you displayed at those times.

What qualities or characteristics would you like to display more? Are they the same qualities that you would like to attract in another? Just know that we attract the same energy as we are sending out.

Visualize yourself radiating out the qualities you would like to attract. Picture yourself with one person (perhaps it is a person you find difficult) and see yourself holding a higher image of the person, encouraging and not judging him or her. Get in touch with the feeling that this evokes inside you. Dwell on that feeling and know that, as you send this out, you also attract it in your own life.

Affirmations

I inspire and motivate all those around me.

I am compassionate, encouraging and non-judgmental.

I help people to be in touch with a higher image of themselves.

I attract helpful people into my life.

I am open to all messages around me that help me on my path.

Feng Shui for Your Environment

This is the area of travel, synchronicity and helpful people. The element is metal. Suggestions here are:

- Pictures of mentors

- Paintings, posters or pictures of spiritual guides or angels

- Anything made of metal

- The colors of gray, silver, pewter, copper, white or black (the adjacent colors on the bagua)

- Round, oval or arched shapes

- Pictures of places you have traveled or want to travel

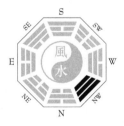

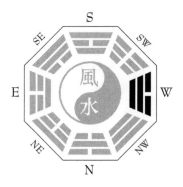

S
SE
SW
E
W
NE
NW
N

CHAPTER 7
CREATiviTY OR OffspsRiNG

Creativity or Offspring Trigram

This trigram, "tui," is represented by a yin line above two yang lines. Because of this formation, the trigram appears outwardly weak but the force and power are within. This is often the case with a lake, one of the meanings of this trigram, where the power is under the surface and the outward appearance is peaceful. The part of the body associated with this trigram is the mouth, which is also where we express the feelings deep inside. In this case, it is referring to joyful feelings, generosity, encouragement and creativity, expressed by the mouth.

On the bagua, it is across from ancestors. It is on the West side of your house. Progeny, creative projects, children or anything we produce depend on where we have been in the past and the lessons we have gleaned from our experiences.

As we work on our creative projects, we refine them as we do metal which is the element of this part of the bagua. In this section, I look at being a parent to our own children as well as to the inner child inside us, educating children, finding creativity and finding the path of joy.

Being a Mother

Usually we take our parents for granted. It is only when we become parents ourselves that we realize how hard a role it is. Yesterday was Mother's Day, and it made me think about growing up with my mother. She is still alive but lives in a nursing home. She has Alzheimer's disease and really doesn't know me any more. Calling her made me sad and started me thinking about early times, growing up with her.

Unlike now, middle class women like her stayed in the home with their children. Where I grew up, it was looked down upon to work when you had children. Women stayed at home and worked around the house and filled their extra time with volunteer and community work. The ones I knew seemed content with their lot and found enough time to get together and do various activities. They did not seem to have the pressures that women have today, such as trying to balance work and family.

Today we, as mothers, feel forced to go to work either because we need the money or because of our own internal pressure to perform. We have learned that we need to compete in a man's world and are learning to act according to the stereotype of a man, but we are also filling the traditional maternal role as well.

As I compare the two roles, I realize that we have lost a great deal. We are dying earlier, we are getting heart attacks, and a lot of the traditional "male" diseases. We are feeling stressed and pressured and often do not take the quality time with our children because we are so preoccupied.

I gave up the traditional role of stay-at-home mother when I left my first husband. I gave up his support and decided that I should venture out on my own. It was scary for me because I was leaving behind the life I knew, the one my mother had led. I was propelled to find something else which was not about having a stable family and money. I believe, in the long run, I have blossomed because of it, but I have often wondered if my children suffered.

When I was young, I would go home from school for lunch and my mother was there to welcome me. I would also find her there when I came home after school. Even if I did not want to talk to her, I knew she was there if I needed her. When small children are growing, they feel more secure in their mother's presence. They venture farther away because they know she is there. When mother is not there, they become more insecure.

When my children were young, I was often not there when they came home. When I was home, many times I was preoccupied and pressured by schoolwork or work and would look after them in a distracted way. I was certainly not there in the way that my mother was for me. She thought that her purpose in life was looking after my sister and me, while I was searching for my purpose.

I think that a great deal has to do with the age that you become a mother. My mother had been teaching for several years and married in her thirties and did not have me until she was 39 years old. She had satisfied her career desires and was ready to settle down and concentrate on family.

Having children, just like education, is wasted on the young. When we are young, we do not know ourselves. We are still trying to find our place in the world and often can hardly look after ourselves, let alone children. The indigenous tribes have it right when they let the elders raise the children. I am a far better mother now.

I compare the two lifestyles—mine with my children and mine with my mother. We, as women, have come a long way in developing our skills but have we lost our connection with people? My mother developed her creativity through arts and crafts and flower arranging. Those skills are not valued much in this world unless we are making money with them.

Which group was happier? I believe that it was my mother's generation and many of them have lived long lives to show it. They might not have been as aware spiritually but many of them lived loving, spiritual lives without understanding the principles. Our generation feels pushed and pressured and nothing is ever good enough. In the last generation, mothers could feel proud of looking after children and did not feel any outside pressure to perform. Many of them would have been wonderful in the business world but did they miss anything by not being there?

What have we gained by being superwomen? We have proven that we can do anything, but how has it developed our relationships or, even deeper than that, our soul? Has it helped us connect with our true purpose?

Because many were forced into the housewife role, the last generation of women may not have connected with their purpose either and ended up feeling very empty. On the other hand, we have many opportunities to work but often our busyness keeps us from connecting to our purpose. What we need is a middle ground, a feeling of fulfillment and the time to reflect in order to know if we are on the right course. One way of knowing is to check with our feelings. Whatever we are doing should feel joyous.

The Path of Joy

How can we handle all our roles and still have joy in our lives? The superwoman phenomenon is often formed from achievement motivation and being conditioned to struggle. You can live your life in many ways on this earth and many of us choose the path of struggle instead of the path of joy. I have talked about the path of struggle in other chapters. How can we walk the path of joy instead?

Are you aware of what brings joy into your life? Do you spend the day doing those things that bring you joy or are you too busy fulfilling daily obligations? Do you live in the present or are you more concerned with how things will be in the future when you can become happy? This part of the bagua is concerned with how we move with joy into the future.

Many of us fill our days with activities that are not joyful, running from thing to thing, feeling harassed and overwhelmed. We think that we will have peace and joy when we have done a certain thing or have made a certain amount of money. We are imagining what it will like to be happy instead of finding present happiness. Happiness, like abundance, is a state of mind to be cultivated in the present. It is present happiness which will bring future happiness.

Finding purpose is doing those things you love to do. You need to find more and more time to do those things daily. Our personality is distracted by things of the senses, as well as the wants and needs of others. We might start the day by wanting to do things aligned with our higher purpose but end up off-course because a phone call, an event, or a situation with another distracts us.

You can choose how you want to live each day even though it does not seem like it. If you are doing work that seems like a struggle and holds no joy, it is time to take another look at that work. Know that life is far beyond what appears on the surface. You will be guided to the work which will bring you joy if you live in the present and look for the synchronicity in all situations.

We are free to choose in every moment. You may have created an area of work based on certain accomplishments and forms. The path of joy is learning not to be trapped by these forms and creations but to be uplifted by them. Like in Feng Shui, if you do not feel energized by them, it is time to change them.

If we could wake up each morning with a higher vision of ourselves and ask how each thing that we are going to do today fits into this vision, we would start to see the path we are to follow. If we can have the courage to eliminate outside distractions and tune within, we are always being given answers from the universe which show us the next step. Sometimes it is phoning someone or meeting an unknown person that can turn our life around.

Often we have less than a joyful existence because we allow people to keep us off course by their demands of us. We somehow feel responsible for them. When that happens, remind yourself that that is old conditioning and your feeling of obligation comes from old messages that we have talked about in other chapters. The path of compassion does not obligate you to be caught up in the dramas of others. We can acknowledge people for who they are, not judge them and know that they have their own path and lovingly release them to follow it.

People who are constantly calling on your energy to help them out of difficulties are draining your energy. When we realize that our help often enables others to stay in their difficulty, we stop and allow them to find their own solutions and rely on us less. The path of joy helps us let go of carrying others.

This path also supports you to give and receive freely and feel grateful for what you have already. When you give, give from your heart and be open to receive what is offered to you. Know that you have been given a great deal already and being grateful opens us up to receive more. As we start to open up and feel joy for even the simple things around us, like birds and flowers, then the universe will send us more joyful things.

When you wake up in the morning, think about what would bring you joy. Instead of thinking about your problems, think about things that make you happy and put a smile on your face. A smile activates the chemicals in your body that make your body healthy.

Create the highest vision of yourself and live it daily. Sit and review your activities and think about whether they bring you joy or obligation. Choose to eliminate the obligations and create your day with joyful activities. As you do this, you will find that a higher purpose of your life will evolve, even if you do not know what that is at this moment.

Your challenge will be to step outside the judgment of others. Other people will not understand what you are doing and will try to steer you off-course by telling you that you should be doing something else. At these times, always go back to your higher vision of yourself and remind yourself that you can choose joy. You are a pioneer on the path and, even though other people may not be aware of it, they may, at a later time, ask you for direction.

Tapping Creativity

Recently, when I threw the I Ching coins and looked up the resulting hexagram, I received "The Well," which is represented by a wooden pole being dipped into the water or a plant drawing water up from the ground. It is to remind us that a town may change but the well remains the same.

How do we get in touch with the well inside of us, the part of us which remains changeless no matter what is going on around us? It appears to me that this part of us is where our creativity originates. We need to connect with that deeper part of ourselves in order to create in our lives instead of react. Most of us are not original thinkers because we do not take the time to sit and contemplate.

We have no peace, and certainly no joy, because we are often in a crisis mode and are fixated on what appears to be going wrong for us. When we are in that state, we cannot access the deeper part of ourselves where we can come up with creative solutions.

Eastern philosophies remind us of the changelessness which exists inside us, the part of us that is always quiet and peaceful. How do we reach the inner well? I believe that Eastern practices help us to reach the Spirit within. They believe in the philosophy that says when you learn to control the body, you can control the mind, and when you learn to control the mind, you allow Spirit to come in.

When we look at the lives of creative people like Edison and Einstein, for example, we find that they attributed their creativity to their connection to that inner stillness. Often they would spend time alone or even have a short nap. Their creative ideas did not come from forcing themselves to think of a solution but from opening up to the flow of universal knowledge. Many of these very creative people would say that they did not know from where the ideas came but they knew that they could not force them.

How can we get in touch with the more creative parts of ourselves and not always be in a reactive mode? I believe that there are certain things we can do. Since these creative "aha" experiences often come from periods of silence, take some time to be quiet or meditate at least once a day. I will suggest ways of making that process easier in Chapter 8. Taking a quiet walk in nature often stimulates creativity.

As suggested in the first chapter, try to live more in the present and go with the flow. The more rigidly attached you are to your point of view, the harder it is to be open to new ideas. We need to let go of our attachment to seeing things in a certain way, knowing that there is always another way. We have to be open to synchronicity in our environment and know that sometimes the answer we are searching for is right there. If we get out of our habitual way of seeing things and try to open up to seeing beyond the normal solution we can become creative, even with problems in our lives. Sometimes, by going off the beaten track, we will run into people who hold the missing piece to a particular dilemma.

Writing in a diary or journal every day will get you in touch with a more creative part of yourself. Sometimes the exercise of writing connects you with a deeper perspective and can be therapeutic. When you review these daily entries, you start to see patterns emerging. As you view this behavior from a more objective viewpoint, you will start changing things in your life. Your dreams are giving you a running commentary on what is going on in your subconscious mind and recording them may give you more insight. If we look at everything in dreams as symbolic, representing a part of us, we can access very valuable information through them. After writing down my dreams and noticing a pattern of chaos and being weighed down, I was able to start letting go of many commitments in my life.

Expect the unexpected and be flexible, knowing that the only thing that is constant is change itself. We sometimes find change difficult, but it is through change that we grow to another level. We need to welcome change, especially changes in our environment. When we try to hold onto things as they are now, we stay stuck in our old conditioning and old

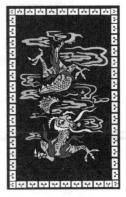

patterns of thinking. We need to release these patterns, in order to be truly in touch with our creativity.

When you are trying to come up with a solution to something, try to think of the very opposite way of handling it from how you would normally do it. That is called contrary thinking and, from that, we often come up with an entirely new solution. This area of the bagua encourages us to get away from our habitual thinking patterns. Even if it against your usual way, try to do just the opposite. When I had my clothing store, I would have people come in who had always dressed in the same style and colors. I would encourage them to get creative and try wearing something entirely different. Often, after they got over their original shock, they liked how they looked and they felt renewed. Sometimes a new look can give you a feeling of more confidence.

Also, you can brainstorm ideas. This is often a good thing to do in a group because you tap the creative juices of many people. In brainstorming, you throw out as many ideas as possible around a given issue. These ideas can be totally "off the wall." The main rule is that you do not judge any of these ideas. It does not matter how wild they are or even how relevant they are to the subject. When I am doing counseling, I encourage people to say anything that comes to their mind without evaluating it first. When we are doing that, we are bypassing the inner censor who is always telling us that this or that is not a good idea. Often very innovative discoveries come out of this kind of thinking. If you look at all the things that we now take for granted, such as cars, trains, planes and even computers, they all were entirely new and original ideas and, when they were first created, were "off the wall."

We can get more in touch with the creative parts of ourselves by taking time to play and enjoy ourselves. This trigram emphasizes our joyous, childlike qualities within.

Often the more child-like we are, the more creative we are. Children are very creative until they pick up the rigid conditioning of society.

Educating Children

Chinese culture believes in educating children in a way that submerges their individuality and makes them an integral part of their group or community. Our culture promotes education that encourages creative individuality and also being a responsible citizen. From what I have observed, we are failing in this educational attempt. We have to remember that our future will be guided by our children. My fear is that we are not giving our children the tools they need to develop in a way that will enhance the future.

Today's children are doing many things which draw attention to them. Some of them are involved in crimes that were unheard of years ago. Many of them are communicating with us but not in a way that we like. In many ways, they are reacting to our lack of direction as a society. They have grown up looking for consistency, love, and respect, but get only confusion and rules that don't make sense. They are searching for a sense of belonging in a community and when they don't find that, they create communities of their own. Many of these communities are based on values rebellious to what they see around them and some are reflecting society's underlying values, even though we would not like to admit it.

Sometimes the crimes, like children shooting other children, shock us out of our apathy and we start to question what kind of society would produce these kinds of offenses. We are more apt to blame the parents or the school system than look at what in our society could foster these extreme actions. Our society is based on violence and war and children see these violent acts committed daily on television or in movies. It is no wonder that they choose violence when they want to resolve some dispute in their own lives.

Having done substitute teaching in elementary, middle and high schools, I see how difficult it is to educate children. With large classes, teachers do not have the time to deal with students individually. As in my childhood, in order to control the classes, there is an emphasis on rigid discipline, rules, and regulations that are not explained. The rules often go against the children's natural instinct to move and talk to other children. Children are treated harshly and told to follow the rules. Some schools remind me of jails with security guards on duty all around.

Children today are more sophisticated and need more explanation of why things are so. The majority of children today need another style of discipline. From a metaphysical viewpoint, these children could have more understanding of why they are here on this planet and feel a deep frustration that they are not more understood.

There is more "attention deficit disorder" than ever before, and many children are being treated by medication. Often this hyperactivity is caused by boredom with what they are learning and how they are being taught. The model of harsh discipline and rules stifles their creativity. The schools that foster the development of the children's individuality and creative processes are having more success.

Home schooling is becoming more prevalent, but is this the answer? The purpose of schooling is not only to develop knowledge, but also to learn to deal with other children of different backgrounds, and to socialize in our society. It is important that children be with other children.

How, then, should we educate children? I believe that children should be honored for who they are, not for what they do. Too often our society's emphasis is on who we are in our occupation and not on who we are as people. "Doing" has become more important than "being." The emphasis in this part of the bagua is on the joy and abandonment of childhood, which we do not allow children to feel very often. Children learn that they will be accepted if they do what their parents want them to do or what is valued in society. Often children are pushed to excel in games and sports. They are often so programmed to win that it is a disaster when they lose. Later they head towards a profession of their parents' choosing, ignoring their own personal wishes and emotions.

Often they deal with the deep dissatisfaction related to not enjoying what they are doing.

If we were all honored for who we are and were allowed to make our own choices, we would have more contentment in our lives. When we punish children, we make them feel that we only love them when they comply with our wishes. It is very important to let them know that we may not agree with their action but we love them nevertheless.

In an ideal society, how would we educate our children differently? In ideal conditions, we would honor each child's individuality and special talents. We would let them express their emotions freely, even anger, and then talk to them, helping them to better understand and work through their feelings.

We would let them know that they were loved and respected and that, in this world, they had a special purpose that only they could fulfill. We would give them encouragement and training to help them fulfill this purpose. We would encourage the development of creativity and let them think for themselves.

We would not leave their care in the hands of the parents alone but have the community at large handle their education. We would let the elderly people pass on their wisdom because, in an enlightened society, it is the elders of the tribe that raise the children. In that type of community, the elders are respected for having lived long enough to see patterns repeat themselves. Children would not be isolated in homes where a chance of abuse exists. They would live in an extended family where they would have support all around. This type of living arrangement is more prevalent in a Chinese society. The Feng Shui bagua shows us that we need the learning of the past for balanced progeny in the future.

Children would be loved, honored and respected in a way that we wish we all could be. We would create boundaries for our children but explain why these boundaries exist. We would explain rules to the children and let them have choices within the rules. When they overstepped a boundary or a rule, they would know the implications and they might even take part in deciding what the consequence might be. Usually a punishment which is meaningful is one which restricts them from doing what they enjoy or a "time out" where they are removed from their usual surroundings to contemplate their behavior.

Physical punishment teaches children that hitting and violence are the way to handle obstacles. In my view, there is never a reason to hit a child. No matter how frustrated a parent might be, it is usually a manifestation of the parent's inability to cope.

Children are capable of making their own decisions and the more we give them a choice, the more self-reliant they will be as adults. We give them the options and the consequences and let them choose. We must always be consistent and when we have made a consequence, it is important that we carry through with it. We allow children their own space but, at the same time, we stay aware of what they are doing. Too much choice sometimes sends them towards the structure of a gang or cult.

Through practices like Qigong and Feng Shui, we would give them practices that calm the body and mind. They would learn not to react to everything going on but to have choices in their reactions. We would teach them focus and balance through some slow movement like qigong and even some meditation. I usually see children who are eternally active, reacting to everything around them and being very easily angered by others' behavior towards them. I would teach them to view life differently and see that others' reactions do not always have to affect them. They would learn to react calmly.

Since I work with a lot of physically and emotionally challenged children, I would have all children spend some time with these children in order to learn compassion and appreciate more their own freedom of movement. I would teach them about all different peoples and cultures so that they learn a broader perspective of their own life.

If we frequently praise our children and encourage all their efforts, as well as respect them for who they are as individuals, we will

114

find that they will grow into self-reliant and confident adults. Most of us wish that we could have had that kind of upbringing ourselves. Since we did not, we need practices that help us work now with the child still existing within us.

FindiNq ThE INNER Child ExERcisE

Most of us are still fighting the child inside us who wants to keep us from moving forward. It is still reacting to past experiences and is afraid to let go. In many ways, it is attempting to keep you safe in the only way that it knows how.

We have developed a sense of powerlessness in our childhood when we were not able to change events easily. Now we do have the power to change things. What we have to be aware of is changing our limiting childhood feelings.

In some cases we need to re-parent our child, knowing that it is still possible to send other messages to our subconscious. What we are doing is reprogramming our mind, replacing the messages that we received in the early years with new empowering messages.

When you are feeling powerless or any strong debilitating emotion, allow yourself to get in touch with this feeling and take yourself back to an early time when you first felt it.

Spend some time journaling or just going within to get in touch with the buried memory which is being triggered. Try to get in touch with that child who still exists within you and really allow yourself to feel the feeling of those times.

After you have delved into these feelings, in your imagination interact with this child, from the vantage pint of who you are now. Give him or her the love and attention that was missing in those early years.

Imagine treating that child as if it were your own child, talking to him or her. Try to really connect with that child and find out what would make him or her happy. What could you do to make that child feel worthwhile and safe?

I have had clients decide to go to the beach, take time to play, or take more time for themselves, getting in touch with the realization that they were not allowed to do these things as children. Visualize a wonderful childhood, bringing in the feelings of joy and happiness.

Affirmations

I allow joy to come into my life.

I am in touch with my creativity.

I nurture my inner child.

I take time for myself and do things that I love to do

Feng Shui for Your Environment

This area is where you emphasize projects, creativity or anything concerning childhood. The element is metal. Suggestions of things to display here are:

- Any projects you are working on
- Pictures of your children
- Any toys or whimsical objects
- Anything round, oval or arch shaped or made of metal
- The metal colors, white or light pastels
- Anything which reminds you of a happy childhood
- Creative objects or art

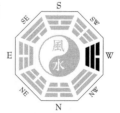

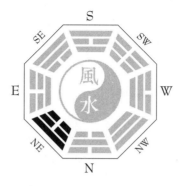

S
SE
SW
E
W
NE
SW
N

CHAPTER 8
INNER KNOWLEDGE

Inner Knowledge Trigram

The trigram "ken" is composed of a solid line above two broken lines, creating the image of space inside something solid, like a cave inside the mountain which is what this trigram symbolizes. The colors are blue and the colors of earth, the element of this trigram. It is on the Northeast side of your house.

The trigram represents a mountain that is static and in repose. For us, this part of the bagua is a time of stillness, a period of waiting and solitude in order to really get to know ourselves. The only way that we can do this is by taking time for contemplation, introspection, wisdom and knowledge. In the archetype of the family, it represents the youngest son.

On the bagua, it is across from the relationship trigram, and both represent the element earth and the qualities of yielding and receptivity. It is through quiet contemplation and inner serenity that we begin to know ourselves. Only through knowing ourselves do we have anything to give in a relationship with others.

In this part of the bagua, we will look at cultivating a quiet mind and going within, finding true power, the meaning of death, dealing with our emotions and finding emotional serenity. The exercise of the healing sounds is given to remove the destructive effects of the emotions on your organs.

Cultivating a Quiet Mind

How do you quiet the mind? If we can become calm and tranquil, we are accessing that part of ourselves that is the deep core, our spiritual self. It is very hard to access because, before we get there, there are lots of thoughts and emotions to wind our way through.

Have you ever been on a vacation and, when you really try to relax, you start thinking about all the things which you have left undone or things that haven't bothered you for years? It is as though all your life is coming up for review. Often you get depressed or you keep doing things that distract you from thinking. When you sit still, everything comes up for you to look at. This also happens in the middle of the night when everything seems disastrous and out of proportion. The more you try to sleep, the more thoughts come to you. Many people resort to taking sleeping pills to escape this constant nagging in their mind.

From the viewpoint of Eastern practices, we strive to get a tranquil state in which we let our thoughts flow through our mind without analyzing or judging them. In Buddhist practices, persistent thoughts are related to the cycle of karma, the things that we have not settled in our past lives, as well as in this lifetime. We need to recognize that they are there, but not get distracted by them.

These practices suggest allowing thoughts to rise and settle in your mind, like the waves in the ocean. They tell us not to grasp or cling to thoughts and not to solidify them. Be like an ocean looking at its own waves. The philosophy is that as your attitude changes and you don't take thoughts as seriously, the whole nature of your thoughts change.

Getting a quiet mind is very much like meditation in that you need to find the place that is the gap between the thoughts. The role of meditation is to allow the thoughts to become farther and farther apart so that gap becomes more and more apparent. Sometimes, if you concentrate on the third eye just above the bridge of the nose, you feel removed from your thoughts.

There are certain techniques that are used in Eastern traditions to be able to quiet the mind. They suggest that you can transform your place of meditation into a sacred space. Use things that inspire you such as readings, poetry, quotations, aromas, or flowers—things that take you beyond your normal mind-set. A good place to meditate is the self-knowledge part of your home.

Our posture is very important. Whether we sit cross-legged on the floor or on a chair, we should sit with our back straight so that the energy can flow smoothly and not get blocked. It is a matter of training our minds and emotions so that we have the control to sit and be quiet whenever we want to—that we are not controlled by outside sources.

There are three methods that are very common to enhance a quiet mind or meditation: watching the breath, using an object, and reciting a mantra. Watching the breath means being aware of breathing while in a relaxed state. When inhaling, breathe in relaxation and, when breathing out, be aware of letting go and releasing tension, frustration, etc. Rest in the natural gap between the in and out breath. Don't concentrate totally on the breath but become more mindful of your breath and of being in the present. Instead of just watching the breath, start to think of yourself as being one with it. The breath is not only calming your mind but it is sending more oxygen to the brain and massaging your digestive organs.

Using an object is another way of focusing your attention. For learning to control the mind and also to improve the skill of visualization, it is a good exercise to concentrate on something like a flower or a crystal. Sometimes gazing at a picture can get you lost in the scene until you lose conscious connection with it.

In a practice called ocular divergence, you stare just beyond an object until you see a blurred vision as both sides of your brain start to blend together. This exercise helps balance the left and right brain so that you are able to access the logical and the creative sides of yourself.

Reciting a mantra or a word over and over again gives you something to concentrate on and takes your mind off your thoughts. In some Eastern practices, a mantra is more than that, however. It is the essence of sound and the embodiment of truth in the form of sound. It can also purify the channels of the body and charge your breath with the energy of the sound.

For example, the mantra Om Ah Hum contains the principal syllables of the Sanskrit language. What is taught is that OM is the fundamental sound behind the cosmos and contains unlimited ability and, in the human body, it is the sound in the head. It sounds like the circulation of the blood and the beat of the heart when you put your hands over your ears. This sound is said to clear the mind, raise the vitality of the spirit and increase wisdom. Om is said to be a short form of "I am," which is the eternal immortal sound.

Ah is said to be a fundamental sound of growth, the first sound made by all life in the beginning, the sound of manifestation. The sound Ah is in the word God in many cultures as in Buddha, Allah, Tao etc. It is also said to open the knots in the body and clear diseases of the organs.

Hum is the sound of the potential of life and the sound of material things. It is the sound in the center of the body, the tan tien. It also opens knots in the channels of energy in the body and helps create health and longevity.

There is a Buddhist Qigong practice that suggests chanting these three sounds with your hands in prayer position. Visualize

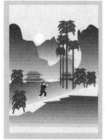

something inspirational in front of you or concentrate on a great light in front of you. Inhale and raise your hands above your head, bringing your hands together, touching the crown of your head and chant OM. Lower your hands down to your throat and chant AH and continue lowering your hands to your heart area and chant HUM.

Research has found that when a person engages in a repetitive prayer, word, sound or phrase, the physiology of our body changes. There is a decrease in blood pressure, heart rate, rate of breathing and slower brain waves. These changes are the opposite of those brought on by stress so these sounds can reduce stress in the body as well.

If we want our lives to go smoothly and demonstrate our purpose, we need to find a new way to handle our everyday existence. We need practices such as these, which can be done daily and even hourly, to remind us of who we are. We need to connect our spiritual life to our daily life and make every thought, word and deed one that represents us on a deeper level.

This kind of behavior takes a deep commitment on our part but, if we do commit ourselves, we start to notice a change in our whole being. How do we do this practically in our lives? For me, the early morning is an important time, the time just after you wake up. If you can take the time, just as you wake up, record your dreams because they are a good indicator of where you are emotionally. Also, if you take the time to think quietly about an issue that is bothering you, as you go to sleep, you will see that you are receiving some kind of answer in your dreams. At first, they may be hard to decipher but, if you keep on recording them, you will find that they start to make some sense, when you go back and read them.

In the early morning, a physical practice like Tai Chi or Qigong will relax as well as energize your body so that you will be resilient and able to handle anything that happens. As we stressed before, these practices emphasize a physical movement which shows you how to handle life—yield, pull back, stand in openness and move only when it is time to move. If you do this enough with your body, it starts to show itself in your life. Something which would have brought a drastic reaction in the past now does not disturb you in the same way.

The other time that is very important to quiet the mind is the time just before you go to bed. It is best to go to bed with as quiet a mind as possible so that, while you sleep, you are open to the spirit realm. Using the practice of the Healing Sounds (given to you in the end of this chapter) helps clear the emotions from the affected organs and balance the body so that you have a better rest.

Just before you go to bed is also a time to stop and reflect on the day's activities. I find journaling is a good idea because, as you write, you often connect with your higher wisdom and develop a deeper understanding of your actions. Also, as I said before, you can reflect on a problem that you are having and ask that you receive guidance in your dreams. You will be amazed at how the solutions start to come to you in your dreams and in creative moments during the day.

We receive messages from our spiritual self daily and, most of the time, we are too busy to hear them. Our old ways of trying hard and thinking deeply about something make our problems more unsolvable. The best thing is to relax and be open to the solutions that we are sent. Trying too hard or worrying sends the solutions away.

During the day, try to take some time to get quiet, even if it is at your desk at work. Some brief meditation, in order to tune out the world, will give you a fresh start and a new perspective. When you are totally embroiled in some challenge or decision, that is the time to pull out, take a walk in nature or just sit and blank out your mind. You start to see that, if you wait, a solution will be given to you.

Many of us already know that this kind of practice would help us in our lives but we still do not do it. We continue to run from place to place and do not find that time. I suggest to you that you make a conscious effort to try it, for at least thirty days, and see if it makes a difference. I guarantee that as you get in the habit of doing this daily, you will miss it when you stop. Try to make it as much of a habit as the daily rituals (like cleaning your teeth and brushing your hair) which you have now. As you start to do this regularly, you will access your inner power.

Inner Power

Power, as the world knows it, means power over something else or power in terms of accumulated goods or material possessions. It means that people are more powerful than us because they have more money, possessions, or greater physical strength. Sometimes it means that we have to give in to the suggestions and advice of others because we see them as being more powerful. Sometimes we have to submit to others' authority in the workplace or even at home because someone else is paying our bills.

All conflict, whether it is between a couple, a family, a community or between nations is a desire for false power. We think that by getting power over someone or something we have won something: wealth or possessions, perhaps. Maybe we think we've won the ability to inflict our values on someone else. In the long run, though, we have won nothing. When we talk about false power, we are talking about anything from the outside which we think will complete us. These can be possessions, money, relationships—even drugs, alcohol, or food.

There is a power that is beyond everything from the outside, one which will give you control over your emotions, mind, body, relationships, health and even your finances. It is power of the Spirit within and it is available to all of us. When we realize that our center of power is our spiritual self and that all of us have this power, our perspective changes.

"The Tao that can be spoken about is not the real Tao," says the *Tao Te Ching*. Inner power is not something that you can see or talk about. I'm sure that you have run into people who have a certain air about them that you cannot describe—you just feel. They may be in a position of worldly power or they may be doing some menial job in the eyes of the world.

The first time I felt this kind of power was when I met an old Native Indian chief who was attending a conference with me. He led a ceremony for us and what was most noticeable was the peaceful countenance of this old man. Later, I found out he lived in a very simple way without possessions.

He sat in a very peaceful, calm manner and spoke of the wisdom of his people who knew how to communicate with nature. As he spoke, there was something emanating from him that was beyond the words he spoke. I will not forget it because it had a very calming effect on me. I was much younger and had a headache at the time, maybe caused by the very intellectual frame of mind I was in. What I felt from him took me by surprise. He was no longer concerned with worldly possessions or being in a position of authority. It was obvious that he took his authority from something else. What I felt was: Why are you bothered with the things that are concerning you? There is something beyond all of those things that is more important and, if you connect with it, it will bring you true peace unavailable in things of the world.

Since that time, I have run into other people with that quiet power, many who are engaged in Eastern practices. The philosophy underlying these practices is based on the premise that we are spiritual beings having a sojourn on earth and that our real power is based in the spiritual world or in the Tao.

When you think of this in terms of power, does it mean that you give up your power to a higher authority just the way you give up worldly power? Giving up worldly power to someone else means letting another person make decisions for you and putting your destiny in their hands.

In surrendering to Spirit, you lose the feeling of individuality. Surrender here means enlarging your vision to "having to do it all yourself," to aligning yourself to the powerful forces at work in the universe today. The difference is that you are aware of a greater plan of which you are a part. Having inner power means letting Spirit guide you, realizing that you are part of a much grander force, and that you can access this force to do anything you want to do. Inner power, then, is based on who you are as a divine being and connects you to the powerful forces of the universe. Inner power means that you remain strong and confident because you know that real power does not exist at the level of the world.

Worldly power, on the other hand, means power over someone, implying that one person submits to another. Each person is separate and individual, competing with one another. It is based on who you are as a personality, and you can lose this power. Other people can steal your money or possessions, illness can steal your health, and age can take your strength.

In other words, worldly power is based on fear. Fear tells you that you cannot trust people, you have limited resources which you must watch carefully or they will be taken away. You must stay away from germs or you will get sick. Other people will take things away from you. You live in a competitive world and you might not make it. You are afraid that you will lose your job, that you will not get a position, etc.

The more powerless people feel, the more they try to grasp power from others. It is evident in the world through countries that try to dominate and overpower others. Most of the atrocious crimes committed by individuals or nations have been done in the attempt to feel more powerful. But it is an endless struggle because the more power you try to grasp, the more elusive it becomes. There is no end to the power grasping. Even addiction to drugs, alcohol, food, relationships or anything else can be a search for more power, trying to fill our bottomless pit from the outside.

How do we change this endless struggle for power? We take another view of what happens around us because there is always a deeper meaning. It is based on the premise that we are all connected and part of a divine plan, that the divisions that we see between us are of the world but not of Spirit. How do we feel that connection and not get carried away with our everyday activities? There are two Taoist concepts which can help us: non-attachment and non-action.

Non-attachment

As we said before, real power is not of this world. As we try to hold onto things that tend to make us feel powerful like possessions, money and jobs, we see that they bring us no peace. The more we have, the more we want and the harder it is to keep it.

Even if we have possessions, the more we remain detached from them, the easier it is for us to enjoy them and allow them to come and go. We remain detached from things of the world because we are not sure what anything means. We are obviously not on this earth to take care of possessions or to amass great fortunes. We see what happens to great fortunes of the world as we dig them up from where they became buried eons ago. The purpose of life is not to leave monuments, but to return to our spiritual selves.

Non-attachment is a surrender to Spirit. Surrender does not mean a giving away of our power as we would if we surrendered to something in the world; instead, it is a way of connecting to a power greater than ourselves of which we are a part. Remember the example in Chapter 1 of the ocean and a drop of water of the ocean. If a drop of water thought it was on its own, by itself, it would not make much impact. But that drop of water can be part of the whole which makes it part of a very powerful entity. By itself it can do nothing, but with the power of the force of the ocean behind it, it can literally move mountains. Look at the devastation caused by tidal waves and by water with the force of hurricane winds behind it. In the same way, we are part of a spiritual force.

When we know we are part of this force, we become detached from the importance of the things around us and see them from a greater perspective. Many of the esoteric works available today tell us that we, as human beings, are part of a greater plan, which affects the whole universe. We cannot always know why certain things are happening to us but there is usually a deeper purpose.

How do we detach from situations that have us totally involved—whether they are problems of relationships, money, work or life situations? People always feel that to remain detached means not caring what happens. It does not mean that we remove ourselves from the situation but, instead, we try to see it from a higher and greater perspective, knowing that there is a

lesson to be learned. The more that we worry about it and ruminate over it, the harder it is to come up with a solution.

Sometimes, if we reflect on the situation peacefully, we will get
some feeling about what the pattern is and what the lesson might
be. Then the solution will appear to us. To find that solution, our
old way would tell us to get active and go out and do something.

The spiritual way is the concept called non-action. By this we
mean "being in the flow" as opposed to actively pursuing something.

Non-action

Have you ever been in a situation when something happens
effortlessly without you even trying? It is what athletes call "being
in the zone." It is that state when everything seems to connect
easily without effort. Think back to a time in your life when everything seemed to flow. That is what we mean by non-action.

This type of action is called "acting without doing" which is a
very hard concept for us to understand in our society. It is a different way of viewing the world. Instead of striving for goals, we
are very centered in the now, watching for the synchronicity of
each moment. It means remaining in touch with inner guidance
and knowing when to act and when not to act. If you think about
something important which happened in your life, it may have
taken place without any planning. For example, I never dreamed
of leaving Canada and living in Florida. It was a synchronous
chain of events, as I talked about elsewhere, which brought me
here.

As I also mentioned before, struggling for everything was the
way I was conditioned from my parents. If you did not struggle
for something, it was not worth having. The idea of non-action for
my parents would be laziness and indolence. My father would say
"You can't just sit and contemplate your navel," but that is exactly what you should do. In fact, the Taoist practices believe that
you have a type of brain or center of intuition in the area of your
navel or just below (tan tien). The feeling that we get in our "gut"
or in this center is often our intuition at work.

When we work with that center as our guide, we move effort-lessly and things seem to open up for us. We move when things flow for us and we stop when things are not flowing.

The important thing is to note the difference between reacting to a situation and having your own power. When you are react-ing to a situation, you are pitting your power against something but you are not coming from strength. When you are coming from your own power, you are sure of yourself and your own decisions because they are not influenced by anyone else.

Many times you will be in a situation with another person in which that person doesn't agree with your decision and this per-son could be your spouse or even your boss. You might be mov-ing against the world around you and it takes an inner strength to continue with your decision.

Try to be aware of the difference between inspired intuition and your old conditioned responses. These old responses, typi-cally your first reactions, are usually driven by fear. Inner guid-ance feels wise and joyful and usually comes without much thought. Wait until the fear has subsided and be guided by what feels joyful. Trust your own decisions and try not to be influenced by the opinions of those around you. Others will have a lot to say to you and will try to influence you, but learn to trust yourself to know what is the best course of action for you.

The next section looks at a difficult subject, the meaning of death. Acceptance of death comes with more self-awareness. If faced, it can give you a sense of freedom in your life.

The Meaning of Death

When my sister died, I was 21 years old and could not under-stand why she had died at such an early age (25 years old). It left me thinking that life was not safe and that it was not a good idea to be adventurous. She had a mountain climbing accident in Malaysia, while working in an exciting diplomatic job with the Canadian embassy there. For years after-wards, I was perplexed about the meaning of life because her brief life, although full of accomplishments, seemed to have ended before she had experienced a full existence. The joy left my family's life and we were sad and cautious, afraid to experiment with anything new. I had been planning to visit Mary in Malaysia the following summer but, after her tragic accident, decided to marry and settle down. What I learned, with my understanding at that time, was that I should seek certainty and security as I knew them.

Now that my viewpoint has changed, I look back at her death and know that we had something to learn from her short life. The last time that I spent any real time with her, the year before her death, she was not the jealous, sometimes bad-tempered child that I remember from childhood. She had become more unconditionally loving and inspired me to think about what I wanted to do with my life.

My life had been so tied up with her accomplishments that I was not able to develop outside of her. My parent's lives had so completely revolved around her that it was hard for them to have much time for me. Because her academic, music, and athletic career had been so impressive, it was difficult for me to do anything that would interest them. Their emphasis was on achievement or "doing." I lived very much in my sister's shadow.

Sometimes I believe that she knew that she was going to die at an early age because she accomplished so much and left a favorable impact on so many people in a short time. I remember her remarking about a friend who had died young, that it was a romantic way to go because you would always be remembered in your prime. I believe that her short life left a lasting impression on many people, but was particularly supposed to impact me. She was very interested in many cultures, and her travels in the West Indian islands, coupled with her newspaper writings about them, had influenced me to meet her West Indian friends. Eventually I met my own, and I married a Trinidadian.

She took quite an interest in Malaysia, particularly in the Chinese influence on the culture. After her death, many of her possessions came back to us and there were many Chinese items and artifacts. My interest in Chinese culture was influenced by these things.

Did she leave the world a better place? I believe that, as I said before, she touched a lot of people. Her infectious enthusiasm, brightness and boundless energy were long remembered. Those of us that felt the impact of her death looked at life more deeply.

Anybody who has been in your life briefly and has left it through death has left you with a lesson. Usually it is to view life differently. Instead of taking it at face value, you now realize that there is something beyond what you see. Often children who pass through your life briefly and die early have a message of peace and love. They seem to be old souls and are very loving and caring and you wonder why they have been taken from you so soon. You rail at God and wonder why He could be so terrible as to take away this blessed child.

If you look at life as everlasting and believe that we all are here briefly, we realize that some people have fulfilled their purpose much sooner than others. If we look at purpose from a worldly perspective only, we say that the departed missed out on life. They could have achieved so much more because they had such talent or they should have had the experience of children, family or worldly observations.

We look back at history and we look at those who had power and influence and we decide that the way to impact the world is to leave a legacy. This legacy can be material possessions, money, military victories or political influence. If we look at the spiritual side of our life, we see that, when we leave this earth, we can't take any of our accomplishments with us. Perhaps our legacy is to influence those around us in a positive manner.

Usually the death of people close to us helps us take a deeper view of life and leads us to a more spiritual understanding. This part of the bagua emphasizes that we cannot go forward without this self-knowledge. The esoteric literature reminds us that we go from lifetime to lifetime with certain lessons. We have karmic attachments in every lifetime and we repeat relationships in order to clear up these lessons. The people around us, even briefly, help us to clear these karmic attributes.

The next section deals with another part of our karmic overlay, our emotions and how to deal with them.

Dealing with Emotions

From the time we are children, we feel a great deal of emotions. Some of our strong emotions like anger and sadness are caused by childhood experiences, and other unexplained emotions, like phobias, are probably brought in from other lifetimes. Most of us have learned to repress our emotions from early on. Our parents or early caregivers were uncomfortable with their emotions (as they had been taught by their parents) so they stopped us as soon as we expressed any strong emotion.

We have been taught that as soon as we feel a specific emotion it should be submerged. This can lead to very unhealthy expression of emotions. Unexpressed emotions probably cause many of the psychological problems that have become societal problems today.

There are many classifications of emotions and it is generally agreed that cross-culturally we express the same emotions but, depending on the culture, we show them or repress them under different circumstances. Our natural instinct to express these emotions becomes thwarted when our family and indeed the culture tell us—even indirectly—that we are not to show them or even feel them. It is the repression of emotions that creates many problems of our world. Because of this holding in of emotions, people often develop addictions and many psychological problems. Their relationships with other people become distorted and, at the world level, relationships among nations are rife with wars and other conflicts.

Repressed anger becomes rage, repressed grief becomes depression, repressed love becomes possessiveness, repressed fear becomes terror and panic, and repressed envy becomes jealousy. All these extreme emotions can cause havoc in your bodies, relationships, and in societies in general.

How can we foster the healthy development of emotions? I often work with people who have reached middle age, and their emotions have become somatized in their body. I encourage a healthy expression of old emotions by going into the old situations in hypnosis and reliving some of those early emotions. I am always fascinated by the fact that people tell me about a situation while they are in a conscious state and it does not seem to mean anything to them. Under hypnosis, the same situation can cause extreme emotions that they have repressed all these years. I always encourage them to connect with these strong feelings, always being aware that they can remove themselves from them when it becomes too uncomfortable. When they emerge from this state, invariably they will remark that they had no idea that they felt this way. Some emotions take people back into past life experiences. Sometimes the expression of this emotion acts as a catharsis and helps clear up some of the problems that they have in the present.

Since I blend my Western methods with the Eastern, I also work with processes that remove the repressed emotional toxins from the inner organs. Qigong philosophy believes that there is a link between the emotions and the organs. Certain emotions damage certain organs and, conversely, cultivating certain virtues can heal the damage. In Chinese terms, a virtue means a power that can be cultivated and this power can create health.

Anxiety, sorrow, grief, sadness and depression take their toll on the lungs. These emotions weaken the lungs and interfere with the healthy breathing patterns. The lungs are healed by the Chinese virtue yi, translated as courage or righteousness, a sense of integrity and dignity. Lungs are associated with the season of autumn and the element of metal.

Chronic fear causes diseases of the kidneys, adrenals and lower back. In fact, fear (often felt as stress) can cause secretions of large amounts of adrenaline and hydrocortisone which signal the cells to break down stored fats and proteins into glucose (sugar). This stimulates the body into the stress reaction—the fight or flight syndrome—which, if it becomes chronic, causes the shutting down of growth, repair and reproduction by inhibiting essential chemicals and immune function. In Qigong theory, the kidneys also control memory and brain function and fear and stress can create learning disabilities and can damage memory. When the kidneys are healthy, the feeling is gentleness like calm water, the element associated with the kidneys. The virtue associated is zhi, meaning wisdom and clear perception.

Anger, inappropriately expressed or suppressed, damages the liver and leads to muscular tension and various ailments such as headaches, eyestrain, hemorrhoids and irregular menstruation. The word "bilious" implies a connection between anger and the liver. The positive emotion of the liver is kindness, the Confucian virtue wren, meaning the companionship of a good friendship. The associated element is wood.

Impatience, hastiness, arrogance, excitability, excessiveness or cruelty overstimulate and damage the heart, leading to heart disease as well as insomnia, hysteria and psychosis. The positive virtue of the heart is li, meaning ritual but, more than that, the state of mind required for the ritual, one of sacredness, reverence, love, honor, orderliness and sincerity and the element associated is fire.

Worry, obsessive thinking and preoccupation damage the spleen and its associated organs, the pancreas and stomach, causing gastric upsets, elevated blood pressure, weakened immunity and a tendency towards catching colds. The cultivation of xin, feelings of fairness, openness, acceptance, trust and faith heal the spleen. It is associated with the element of earth and can be balanced by spending more time in nature.

The ultimate aim of both Western and Taoist practices is to feel the emotion but not let it take hold. What we are able to express appropriately does not get repressed, to come out later in a very distorted way or to make us sick later on.

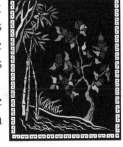

We need practices that both break the loop of repetitive thought which keeps us in that old emotional way of behaving and ones which help us to release the blocks and move the emotion smoothly through our body without taking hold. I introduce one of these practices in the next section.

Six Healing Sounds

I am giving you these very powerful exercises with the permission of Mantak Chia, who introduced to the West these Taoist practices which help release buried emotions from the organs. The position for all these movements should be in a upright sitting position on the edge of a chair with your feet flat on the floor. The sounds should be repeated three times or any multiple of three. When this emotion is causing you a problem, repeat it many times. You will find relief.

Lung Sound

This is to relieve the lungs from any buried sadness, grief or depression. As you become aware of your lungs, take a deep breath and raise up your arms slowly so that your palms are facing your body. When they reach to the top of your head, turn your hands so that the palms face upwards and extend them above your head. Look up through the space in your hands. As you exhale, you put your teeth together and say the sound "SSSS" like a snake sound. As you say the sound either out loud or under your breath (subvocally), imagine that you are releasing sadness from your lungs. When you have let all your breath out, gently bring your hands back to your lap. Now smile into your lungs and imagine a beautiful diamond white covering them and concentrate on the positive virtues of courage, righteousness, surrender and letting go.

Kidney Exercise

Start again with your hands on your lap and focus on your

kidneys. Place your legs together with your ankles and knees touching. As you bend forward, take a deep breath and hold onto your knees, one hand holding the other one. Straighten your arms so that you can feel a pull at your lower back where your kidneys are located. As you exhale your breath, make the sound "WOOO," like the wind in the trees or like blowing out a candle. At the same time, pull in your stomach and imagine that you are releasing any buried fear from the kidneys. When you have exhaled, focus on the kidneys and imagine them covered with a bright, dark blue light and concentrate on the feeling of gentleness. When you have fully exhaled, open your legs again and put your hands palm up on your legs.

Liver Exercise

Sit again in the upright position, your hands resting on your lap. Become aware of your liver on the right side under your diaphragm. Put your hands out to the side, palms up and bring them slowly up until they are over your head where you clasp them and turn them over so that your palms face the ceiling. Bend slightly to the left, so that there is a gently pull on the right side where your liver is located. Exhale the sound "SHHHHH," like telling someone to be quiet. Imagine that with that sound you are releasing all anger from your liver. As you finish exhaling, imagine your liver a bright spring green and focus on the feelings of kindness.

Heart Exercise

The heart exercise is done exactly the same way as the liver exercise except that you lean to the right stretching the left side or the heart area. As you exhale, the sound is "HAWWWWW" and, as you say this sound, you can imagine releasing impatience, anxiety, arrogance and hastiness. Imagine a bright red covering the heart and feel love, sincerity, respect and honor.

Spleen Exercise

Take a deep breath and lean forward, placing the fingers of your two hands together with the backs touching. Place these fingers, like a knife, slightly under the left of the sternum. Press in with the fingers as you push our your back. As you exhale, the sound is "WHOOOOO," similar to the kidney sound but more guttural. As you exhale, imagine getting rid of excess worry. Come back to the sitting position and see the spleen and the associated organs, the pancreas and stomach, covered with a deep golden yellow and concentrate on the feelings of fairness, compassion and trust.

Triple Warmer Exercise

This refers to the three energy centers of the body. The upper level, which consists of the brain, heart, and lungs, is considered hot. The middle section with the liver, kidneys, stomach, pancreas and spleen is considered warm and the lower level with the kidneys, bladder, and sexual organs are considered cold. This exercise is meant to balance the temperature of these three levels of the body. This one is done lying down on your back. Close the eyes and take a deep breath. As you exhale, imagine that a big steamroller is pressing out your breath starting at the top of your chest and ending at your lower abdomen as you say the sound "HEEEEEE." Imagine your body temperature balanced. This is a wonderful exercise to help you go to sleep at night.

These exercises help release emotional blocks from your body, either from the present or buried from past experience. At bedtime they remove the tensions of the day and help you have a restful sleep.

Affirmations

I release all emotional blocks.

I take quiet time for contemplation every day.

I flow with my emotions and allow no emotion to

damage my body.

Feng Shui for Your Environment

This is the area of your house to emphasize quiet contemplation and self-knowledge. The element is earth. Suggestions are:

- A shelf of books
- The colors of blue or the earth tones
- A quiet sitting space for contemplation
- Pictures of mountain scenes
- Anything that reminds you of inner knowledge, meditation or contemplation

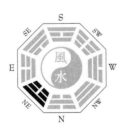

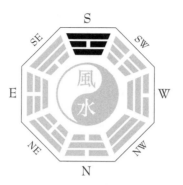

CHAPTER 9

MASTERY

Fame Trigram

The trigram for fame, "Li," is represented by a yin line between two yang lines. Like fire, the element of this trigram, it looks firm and unyielding on the outside but, in fact, is hollow inside. In the archetypal family, it is the middle daughter. The color is red like fire and it encompasses all the characteristics of fire (brightness, heat, and dryness). This trigram is called fame but it is not worldly fame but illumination—how we shine our light and become a master. It is how we are known to others not in the worldly sense, but how our inner being is displayed to others.

In the bagua, it is across from journey. It is on the South side of your house. As we journey through life, we reach self-realization and display our authentic selves to others. Even though we achieve some worldly fame, it is more important to honor our purpose as we pass through our earthly journey. In this area, I look at our own illumination, sounding our note, what we can learn from natural disasters and how we become a master in our own right.

Illumination

Be the light that you are here to be. "By your works are you known," says the Bible. Our fame and reputation are the way we walk in the world. Does that mean that we have to try to be perfect all the time? No. But it means that we have to be honest about who we are, examining ourselves on all levels and working at releasing old patterns that are holding us in behavior that no longer serves us.

This area of the bagua is represented by fire, illumination. Fire lights up everything around us and it also is a bright, sustaining energy that burns briskly and then goes out. It is important not to let our fire go out. When we speak of fire inside of someone, we refer to that quality that represents consistency and power.

In businesses, the "fire" departments are the sales and marketing that sustain the company and keep it going. Likewise, the fire inside us needs to sustain us and keep us going. When we feel that consistency, others feel it, too.

Our light is demonstrated in every action. When we have truly examined ourselves, our actions are in accordance with who we are. When we hold onto emotions—if we are spiteful, bitter, or jealous, for example—we have many unexamined parts. When we get more in touch with ourselves, we feel our emotions, express them appropriately, and release them.

Our integrity will go before us. By integrity, I mean being authentic in our behavior. Whatever we believe in, we must show it through all our actions, not just our words. We need to take the path of honesty, no matter how that may affect us. Sometimes, the more expedient shortcut for us might be to engage in some dishonest behavior. We think that it really won't matter because no one will know. When we are truly aware, we know that every action matters and everything we do returns to us.

One of the aspects in which we will be known is our ability to show unconditional love. This type of love has no agenda and has no expectations of people. We simply accept people the way they are with no qualifications, always seeing the highest image of them, even if they don't see it for themselves. People often feel better about themselves in our presence, even if they have no idea why.

When we are truly a light, we burn with a consistent flame that brings consistency into everything around us. It is hard to feel that steadiness in this world when many things appear to be chaotic around us. However, the more consistent that we feel, the more we create this in the world around us. When we give up the need for chaos in our lives, we attract more peaceful situations.

We start to adopt the mind-set that everything in the world happens for a reason. It is there to show us the parts of humanity which remain unhealed. Even the death and destruction evident in much of what we see and read about in the papers are showing us the group consciousness that surrounds us.

For eons, the human race has been demonstrating chaos and confusion as it holds onto old destructive patterns. According to the spiritual literature of many cultures, this is the lifetime to release these patterns. Sometimes we look around us and think that our contribution can't mean anything because it would be such a drop in the bucket.

If each of us starts to feel and act differently, we are combining our light and can change the world. It will take a ground swell of enough people to reach a critical mass at which time everything, including laws and governments, will change.

Do not ever believe that what you do won't matter. One person exuding light which is full of love has more far-reaching influence than you would ever believe. Several people holding on to a consistent image and sending light can change the world.

By changing the world, I don't mean forcing people to think the way you do but holding a higher picture of humanity, knowing that it is capable of much more than has been demonstrated in the past. Showing our light means being in touch with the power within and radiating it out.

Sounding Your Note

This is the name of a channeling by Orin that I find very helpful. It guides us to evoke our soul essence which has a note or a frequency uniquely our own. When we are able to calm our outer self or personality, we are able to sense, if not hear, this note, in order to project it out so that we attract the people who are to work with us or be with us this lifetime.

As we release blocks in all areas of our lives, we become aware of our higher purpose and we start to have people appear that somehow connect with this. It does not matter what we are doing in the world of work. Our purpose may be demonstrated through our work or it may be in the hobbies and other activities we like to do. We radiate out to the world our authenticity and how it connects with how we spend our time. As we clear the blocks in our lives and relationships, our right livelihood will find us.

The contradiction in all of this is the more we let go and work with the Tao or Universe, the more we find our purpose. It is the opposite of what the world believes. It is not developing the "doing," but the "being." We can't try to do this because trying is the opposite concept of just allowing ourselves to be.

We are clearing away our worldly perceptions and, as we get more in touch with ourselves as souls with a higher purpose, we realize that we have a message to give to the world. As we discover this peaceful way of living, we will want to share it with others. We may do it through workshops, writing, speaking, art or simply by influencing people by our presence.

One of the hardest places to do this is in intimate relationships because, as has been pointed out, these bring up for us all of our old patterns. To know ourselves as spiritual beings, we have to look at how we are functioning in our relationships. If we still are embroiled in conflicts or petty grievances we are not working at a deeper level.

The way to get in touch with our higher purpose, soul essence, or light is to see it in another. The hardest thing is to see it in another when they are not aware of it themselves. When the people around us are buried in dysfunction, we have to be aware of their higher presence and project it for them. This is very hard to do when they touch us with the same old emotional buttons. One sign that we have arrived is that we don't react with the old knee jerk reactions. We may feel them but we see through them.

We recognize that these patterns don't serve us any more and we let them go.

When something someone says makes us react strongly, we know that part of us is not healed. If we feel insecurity, anger or fear, we know that our inner child is still not healed. As we said before, we don't repress it for it to fester, but we acknowledge it, asking that the child within help us in our new understanding. We have a lot of options that we did not have before. Just remember that it does not matter how often these old emotions surface. What matters is that we are able to work through them.

Getting in touch with our soul essence is, I believe, why we are on the planet this lifetime. We get so bogged down by the world and problems that we not do take the time or have the presence of mind to put things in perspective.

As we get more into this philosophy, as demonstrated in Eastern practices, we simply yield, detach and move with the flow of life, knowing when to move simply by an inner knowing, not anything from the outside. We become the movement of the Tao. Nothing will move us off center because we will know that it has a higher purpose.

The Lesson of the Hurricane

Most of us have plans for our days and we know what we are supposed to do from minute to minute. We are so tied down to these plans that we do not take time to listen to any type of guidance or be aware of synchronicity in our environment.

I became very aware of this fact again when I was faced with preparations for an impending hurricane. I had several things to do and was planning for a trip to Trinidad and had appointments set up on the day of my arrival. When the radio announced that there might be a hurricane coming to Florida, I had my mind completely set on leaving town. It was annoying to think that the weather might cause me to change my plans. Instead of getting ready for my trip, I would have to spend my time preparing my house (an arduous process of putting up shutters and removing all items from outside) and running out to get water and canned goods in case of power shutdowns for days. My flight was also canceled and I had to call Trinidad and change all my appointments.

What was that about? When I got through my initial annoyance and took the time to be quiet, I started to contemplate the fact that we never really know what we are going to do from moment to moment. We know what we would like to do but we must always be open to change. We can have some idea of where we would like to end up but often we are not sure of the way to get there.

As we become more aware of our own mastery, we become more cognizant of the partnership that we have with the divine part of ourselves. This part, I believe, is connected to a master plan of the universe and we are moving with this when things go smoothly and start to flow for us.

When earthquakes, hurricanes or other natural disasters come into our lives, we are reminded that things are not as they seem on the surface. We get so caught up in our worldly concerns that we do not take the time for the spiritual side of ourselves. Our earthly possessions may be destroyed but we, as spiritual beings, are not affected. Even though it is hard to remember this fact, surrounded by earthly reminders, our identity is not through these things but through our spiritual understanding.

How would masters handle something like a hurricane or earthquake? They would know that a disaster is in their lives for a reason and they would get quiet and ask to be shown the purpose. Masters would remain watchful and be open to any signs that would show the meaning of the storm and move with the disaster, not against it. They would remain peaceful, visualizing a peaceful outcome to whatever is presented at the moment. They would know that a spiritual view of a peaceful outcome might not necessarily be the same as the world would view it. They would know that there is always a solution to every problem, as dire as it may appear to be.

This is a model to handle all problems that are presented in your life. The first quality that is important is non-judgment because, as we noted before, we never know why problems are in our life. There are always lessons to learn and, if we walk through the challenge ignoring the lesson, we will have these things presented to us in another form. As I have shared, I have gone through many lessons, financial and otherwise, many times before I learned the lessons, took back my own power and create a different reality.

As you start to acknowledge your own responsibility in the creation of these problems in your life, you will be ready to change some of the patterns that keep creating the same circumstances over and over again. At a deeper level, you are aware that you created these problems in order to find the solution and become more enlightened. This is a hard thing to keep uppermost in our mind but, when we do, our life is more joyous and flows easier. As well as non-judgment, we also can remain non-attached to the outcome of events and even to what is happening around us, knowing that we are part of a spiritual universe. We remind ourselves that everything around us is simply giving us a message and nothing is as it seems.

When we are truly walking on the path of mastery, holding our light, we are living our true purpose here. As absorbed as we may be in events of the world, we have to remind ourselves why we are really here. It appears to me that there is a grand design to this universe of which we are only a part and our daily actions need to be reminders of that fact.

In everything we do, we need to shine the light for others who cannot see as clearly as we do. In doing this, we start to be peaceful with ourselves and lose the fear of the unknown. We are truly on the path of mastery.

Becoming a Master

One of the ways to keep on our path is to try to envision being a master or, if that is too difficult, to imagine how we would be acting if we were masters.   What would be different about how we lived our day?

If we think about great masters—whether it is Jesus, Buddha or Lao Tzu—we observe that they moved with a serenity of purpose in which they did not concern themselves with what anybody thought about what they were doing. They knew at a very deep level why they were here, and their thoughts, words, and actions were aligned with that level of understanding.

How can we do this in the present world when we are barraged by so much going on around us? How can we move with the serenity of a master?   I admit that it is difficult, but not impossible.

Once we are more aligned with our purpose, we would give up all the things which did not further this purpose. We would follow the "be, do, have formula" and first be the master in order to do the things aligned to our purpose and have the things that go along with that.

I always ask myself, "How would masters act in this situation?" Masters would not be moved by anything from the outside. Their happiness would not depend on anything but their inner being. In a situation that is challenging, ask yourself what you are to learn from it. What parts of you remain unhealed? Then send healing to yourself and know that you have the power to move past these challenges.

When you get up in the morning, ask yourself how a master would go through the day. A master would wake up with the certainty of purpose and know that whatever needed to be done would be revealed. A master might have plans but would know that these plans could change at any time. Most of all, a master remains confident that inner guidance will show where to go and what to do.

When I move with that inner knowing, I know that people sitting beside me have some information to impart to me or I have something to say to them. I know that everything that happens to me during the day has some higher meaning. I do not worry about anything because I will be shown where I need to be. I will stop pushing myself to do certain things if

145

they do not flow. That is another way that we can know that we are on the right path. When we start to do things and they do not flow, we are probably pushing too hard. When you try something and it is easy to do, it is part of your purpose.

When we are walking as masters, we are feeling calm and certain in our self, knowing that everything is part of a divine plan and that we are part of that plan. We do not allow situations and things to catch us off guard. We do not compare ourselves to people and we are not influenced in any way by people's opinions. Even when something appears to be a problem, we know that the solution is there if we become open to it.

When I find myself worried about something or pulled off center by a situation, I ask myself, "What would a master do in these circumstances?" I imagine an ancient Chinese master, sitting serenely letting the world pass him by, not getting caught up in anything. The *Tao Te Ching* reminds us, "Empty your mind of all thoughts. Let your heart be at peace. Watch the turmoil of beings, but contemplate their return... Immersed in the wonder of the Tao, you can deal with whatever life brings you, and when death comes, you are ready."

Becoming a master means having that inner knowing that you have a purpose for being here and you are here on earth to connect with this purpose. If we rush around doing things, worrying about people and situations, we lose our center and react to everything around us. We do not leave ourselves open to clues in our environment that tell us which way to proceed and what to do.

We are walking in mastery when we can sit back quietly and wait for messages, urges, and feelings that guide us to our next move. A master would wait for the solution to appear, knowing confidently that it will. Sometimes the best thing to do is nothing at all, that status of non-action that we talked about earlier.

Masters know why they are here and would do everything with that inner confidence. We need to remind ourselves that we do have a purpose and, if we move with the flow of life, not against it, we will find that our actions all are joyous and we feel connected to who we are as a deeper being. When you feel weak and uncertain, it is because you have started to doubt this presence within you. When you move with the strength of the universe, you walk in dignity and self-confidence, in humility, not in arrogance.

The path to mastery is to master ourselves. When we have walked through our demons in all areas of our lives, as represented in the Feng Shui bagua, and have connected with our higher presence, we can have full confidence that we are uncovering the mastery that already exists within us.

BECOMiNq A MASTER EXERCISE

Imagine spending a day as a master. Sit quietly, close your eyes and visualize yourself going through a day, starting from the time that you get up in the morning. Imagine this as your most ordinary day, but this time you are going to visualize yourself handling each occurrence as a master would handle it.

See yourself getting up in the morning. Probably, as a master, you would spend some quiet time going within or meditating, setting the tone for the day. As the day progressed, you would move quietly and confidently from event to event without getting upset about anything. As each circumstance happened, you would know that things are not as they seem and that there was some purpose behind everything. You would interact with others in a caring, compassionate way, acknowledging people's higher selves and higher purpose. You would know that they might have some purpose in your life.

If people wanted you to get caught up in chaos or drama, you would not participate nor would you intervene, allowing them to receive their own lessons. You would always be there to remind them of their higher purpose, nothing more.

When things did not work as expected, you would not try to push anything, knowing that there is probably another way to proceed. You would be in touch with higher guidance and intuition at all times and follow it. You would not get frustrated, but instead look for the synchronicity in all situations and try to stay detached from any particular outcome. You would stay still and know when to move, in the true spirit of non-action.

At the end of the day, you would again get quiet or meditate, acknowledging your higher presence and connecting with this presence as you went off to sleep. You would ask for solutions to problems to appear in your dreams.

Now breathe in and see yourself, in your imagination, moving like a master, calm, centered and balanced, knowing that there is something beyond this worldly reality which is more important.

Affirmations

I stay in touch with intuition and inner guidance.

I move with certainty and mastery.

I am a light and I radiate light to all around me.

I am a master.

Feng Shui for Your Environment

This is the area of fire, light, illumination and fame. Suggestions for this area are:

- Anything in the color red or other fire colors

- Candles and lights

- Anything which acknowledges who we are

- Awards or articles on something we have done

- Pictures of animals or people, since animals and people are considered fire

- Fireplaces or fire symbols

- Anything triangular or cone shaped

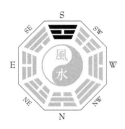

Some Closing Thoughts

I hope that my own experiences have helped you locate blockages in your own lives and that I have given you some tools to be able to clear them away. Using the Feng Shui bagua as a model has helped me become aware of all areas of my life as well as my environment.

This book can be read straight through or it can be used as a divination tool. Through the power of synchronicity, you can open the book randomly and you will find that the section you read somehow connects to a situation in your life. I wish you all the best on your journey to mastery.

WORKSHOPS AND PRODUCTS

CONTACT Dr. Kathryn Mickle for
TELEPHONE COUNSELING, COACHING AND CONSULTATION
The Wellness Institute for Research and Education
2430 Nassau Lane, Fort Lauderdale, Florida 33312
www.thewellnessinstitute.com • email: kmickle@gate.net
(954) 791-2865 • Fax: (954) 791-7358

PERSONAL COUNSELING

"For almost thirty years, I have helped people deal with personal and relationship problems in a variety of ways.

As a therapist, family mediator and practitioner of Eastern philosophy and disciplines, I will help you to break through self-defeating behaviors and find more self-love, deepened inner powers, calm and complete management of your life and strengthened, more loving relationships."

BUSINESS COACHING

"From my years of experience in owning and managing different types of businesses including a retail store, a boat charter business and a seminar and consultation business, I can help you streamline your career. I have found that the secret to success is finding your own key to greatness. I will work along side of you to help you find your purpose, increase your ability to produce results and achieve your maximum potential."

FENG SHUI CONSULTATION

"I have been studying the ancient art of Feng Shui for many years and have found in it, the secret of achieving balance and harmony in my own life. Based on the understanding of the dynamic flow of energy, this practice harmonizes your environment. When you arrange your home or office according to Feng Shui principles, you will be amazed at the dynamic changes in all areas of your life."

FREE INITIAL E-MAIL CONSULTATION

WORKSHOPS AVAILABLE
AT YOUR LOCATION OR OURS
kmickle@gate.net

UNLIMITING YOURSELF

Create the lifestyle of your dreams. Break through barriers and limitations for increased satisfaction and personal and professional success.

JOURNEY TO MASTERY

Learn how to identify and move through blocks in all areas of your life. Learn powerful techniques and tools which help you release limitations and launch you on your journey to mastery.

BUILDING RELATIONSHIPS

People with strong relationships live longer, happier and healthier lives. Examine and move past the blocks holding you back from developing strong, fulfilling relationships.

POWERFUL KEYS TO NEW VITALITY

Time-tested personal development tools from Asian traditions help you to increase health and well being, reduce stress, handle problems effectively and make changes easier.

AN EASTERN APPROACH TO WESTERN CHALLENGES

Blend body, mind and spirit using cross-cultural strategies to reduce stress. Utilize Eastern methods to work through stress blocks and learn coping skills and techniques that calm the body and mind at will.

BASIC FENG SHUI — THE PURSUIT OF BALANCE AND HARMONY

This workshop introduces the principles of Feng Shui and teaches how to balance any environment. These principles help you enhance your career, build your prosperity, solidify your relationships and ensure good health.

PRODUCTS BY AUTHOR

UN-LIMITING YOURSELF VIDEO

This mind-releasing journey will help you eliminate destructive thinking as it power-fully leads you towards more self-love, deep-ened inner powers and strengthened, more loving relationships. The uniqueness of this tape is the blending of beautifully-spoken, healing dialogue with colorful, multi-layered imagery and shaped sound.

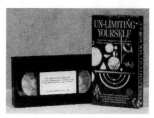

Retail Price $24.99

UN-LIMITING YOURSELF AUDIO

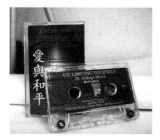

The driving side of this tape, accompanied by up-beat music and drumming, helps you to react calmly to all situations. The medita-tion side, for guided meditation or pre-sleep, uses hypnotic suggestion and music to help you release your limitations and become your strong, powerful, unlimited self.

Retail Price $9.99

TAO CARDS

Bring inspiration and peace of mind into your life t h r o u g h t h e ancient wisdom of the Tao interpreted for the 21st century. Choose a Tao Card, read the inspired message in the accompanying book and allow it to guide you. These cards have been created so that you can choose one a day, one a week, or whenever you need guidance with a specific problem. Discover the impact of ancient Chinese phi-losophy on your modern lifestyle.

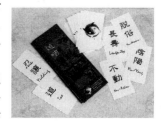

   "This is an attractive set and should appeal to the fans of divination cards, as well as follow-ers of the Tao." — Deepak Chopra's *Infinite Possibilities, Vol. 1, Issue*

Retail Price $29.95

FENG SHUI PRODUCTS

LOVE AND PEACE T-SHIRTS

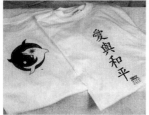

Wear a T-shirt designed with Chinese symbols of Love and Peace. On the back of the shirt is a Yin/Yang logo of two dolphins jumping. As you wear this T-shirt, it is our hope that you will experience and pass onto others the message of the symbols. *Retail Price — $14.95 M & L*
$19.95 XL

FENG SHUI AUSTRIAN CRYSTAL BALLS

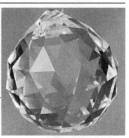

These multi-faceted Austrian Strass crystal balls energize and bring Qi into your home and office. These beautiful prisms bring rainbows of color through your room and balance your environment.

Retail Price $15.00

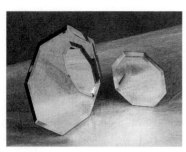

OCTAGONAL DISPLAY MIRRORS

Use these "aspirins" of Feng Shui to draw in positive energy and expand, reflect and strengthen any area.

Retail Price $ 8.00, small
$10.00, large

FENG SHUI WIND CHIMES

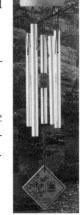

Wind chimes disperse interior and exterior Qi in a more beneficial, balanced way. They assist in bringing prosperity and abundance, balance and harmony into your life. *Retail Price $17.00*

All products available through
The Wellness Institute for Research and Education
2430 Nassau Lane, Fort Lauderdale, Florida 33312
www.thewellnessinstitute.com • email: kmickle@gate.net
(954) 791-2865 • Fax: (954) 791-7358